"This is a great book...necessary reading for not only the victims of cancer, but for the physicians or partners or close friends of those who are afflicted. I certainly would have kept a shelf full of Amy Givler's books and given copies to many of my patients. She has been able to put herself in the position of almost anybody who first hears the dreaded word 'cancer' applied to themselves."

—**Dr. Paul Brand**
Internationally honored orthopedic surgeon and coauthor of *Fearfully and Wonderfully Made*

❧

"While I hope you won't need this book, I'm glad this book is here for you to read. It's like getting a 'house call' from one of God's special physicians who's been there, done that, and knows how God can help throughout it all."

—**John Trent, Ph.D.**
Author, speaker, and president, StrongFamilies.com

❧

"Dr. Amy is a double expert. Not only a knowledgeable physician, she is a cancer survivor. I highly recommend *Hope in the Face of Cancer* to anyone beginning their own journey."

—**Diane M. Komp, M.D.**
Professor of Pediatric Oncology Emeritus, Yale University School of Medicine, and author of *Why Me? A Doctor Looks at the Book of Job*

"In this book Dr. Givler has done an excellent job using her own experience to help people who are newly diagnosed with cancer—providing guidance and helpful information. I particularly like the way she tells the stories of a wide range of people who have coped with a cancer diagnosis."

—Diane S. Blum, ACSW
Executive Director of Cancer Care, Inc.

❧

"Wow, what insight! I wish someone could have put Dr. Givler's book into my hands when I walked out of the doctor's office after hearing my diagnosis. Her book offers solid emotional, medical, and spiritual guidance—in a way that's understandable and not overwhelming to someone who's just heard such difficult news."

—Emilie Barnes
Bestselling author and speaker

❧

"Dr. Givler has written the right book that addresses the right time with the right advice—when the diagnosis of cancer is first heard.

"I strongly recommend this singularly valuable book. It keys into the critical time point when clear thinking is so important to ensure the best outcome."

—Jimmie C. Holland, M.D.
Chair, Department of Psychiatry and Behavioral Sciences, Memorial Sloan–Kettering Cancer Center

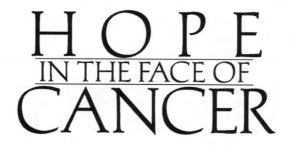

HOPE
IN THE FACE OF
CANCER

AMY GIVLER, M.D.

HARVEST HOUSE™ PUBLISHERS

EUGENE, OREGON

Cover design by Koechel Peterson & Associates, Inc., Minneapolis, Minnesota

Back cover photo: Leslie Arnott

Photo on page 191: Alison Taggart-Barone

Advisory

Readers are advised to consult with their physician or other medical practitioner before implementing any ideas that follow. This book is not intended to take the place of sound personal medical advice or to treat specific maladies. Neither the author nor the publisher assumes any liability for possible adverse consequences as a result of the information contained herein.

HOPE IN THE FACE OF CANCER
Copyright © 2003 by Amy Givler, M.D.
Published by Harvest House Publishers
Eugene, Oregon 97402

Library of Congress Cataloging-in-Publication Data

Givler, Amy, 1958-
  Hope in the face of cancer / Amy Givler.
    p. cm.
  Includes bibliographical references.
  ISBN 0-7369-0990-7 (pbk.)
  1. Cancer—Patients—Religious life. 2. Cancer—Religious aspects—Christianity. I. Title.
  BV4910.33.G58 2003
  248.8'6196994—dc21   2002010023

Printed in the United States of America

03 04 05 06 07 08 09 10 11 12 / DP-MS / 10 9 8 7 6 5 4 3 2 1

To my husband, Don—

a superior doctor,
a wise advice-giver,
a steady leader,
a godly man,
and my best friend.

Acknowledgments

I deeply appreciate all the people who helped bring this book into existence. My husband, Don, and my children, Martha Grace, Pete, and John, contributed in countless ways.

Thanks also to the people who gave practical and moral support, especially Phyllis Alexander, Lesley Arnott, Renee Broyles, Eileen Horner, Madge Huff, Isabelle Middendorf, Tim Nance, Ranga and Uma Rangaraj, Debbie Wallace, Mark and Jennifer Wallace, Brent and Anne Wallace, and my Christian Writer's Fellowship International online support group.

Thanks to Carl Freter, M.D., and Marshall Leary, M.D., for providing a model of what good oncology care looks like.

For helping me hone my writing skills and make my way through the editorial maze, I thank Marlene Bagnull, Elaine Wright Colvin, Paul Gossard, Nick Harrison, Carolyn McCready, Andy Scheer, John and Elizabeth Sherrill, and Monte Unger.

And I give a special word of thanks to the people with cancer whose stories I share in these pages and to their family members. Thank you for being willing to be vulnerable for the sake of others who are just starting out on their cancer journey.

A Personal Word from the Editor

Dear Reader—

On a dark January evening 15 years ago, I walked out of the doctor's office. I had just heard the words, "You almost certainly have some kind of lymphatic cancer."

If only someone could have put this book in my hands back then! I would have been better prepared for the path that suddenly lay before me.

Now, as a cancer survivor, that's why I believe in this book. Its pages are full of hope and full of solid guidance—medical, emotional, relational, and spiritual—that will not overwhelm you. And Dr. Givler has earned the right to give this guidance. First by the profession she chose, and more important, by walking the road she did not choose—the same road on which you or a loved one may now be starting out.

Thank you, Dr. Givler, for writing this book.

Paul Gossard
Editor, Harvest House Publishers

CONTENTS

The Book I Wanted

❧

THIS IS THE BOOK I WANTED when I was first diagnosed with cancer. I remember arriving at our public library within 24 hours of being diagnosed, looking for a book written by someone who had walked this path before me. I wanted to know the path was "walkable," and I needed advice on how to avoid stumbling.

I sat in front of the computer screen, preparing to look up "cancer" in the catalog. Suddenly I looked around to make sure no one was watching me. In my small city, a friend might also be in the library. Typing in those six letters seemed so final—so incriminating—like admitting to the world that I really had this disease, when I didn't even want to admit it to myself.

Finally I chose "Subject," and typed "cancer." Five pages of choices came up. I felt smothered—I felt like I was drowning.

I started over, choosing "Title," then "cancer." Now two books appeared, so at least I could find the right shelf. I went to the stacks and chose five books intended for people newly diagnosed with cancer, and then I rushed out of the library. I didn't want to see anyone I knew who might ask "What's new with you?" I wasn't ready to be truthful.

Once home, I searched the books for an emotional anchor—a way to make sense of what was happening to me. I needed to make intelligent decisions and not just be swept along, overwhelmed.

It was as if I'd taken one step onto a rickety bridge over a gaping chasm—and now I yearned to hear a voice from the other side calling back to me, "I've made it, and you can too!" I wanted those books to give me that kind of encouragement.

They didn't.

Instead, I found too much information—information on what might have caused my cancer, information on what kind of treatments I might expect, as well as extensive information on other kinds of cancer and their treatments.

I had left the Land of Health and had to cross the rickety bridge over the chasm called Cancer. I didn't want to be on that bridge, but the way back was blocked. I couldn't make the cancer disappear.

Who else had crossed that bridge? Could they guide me?

In those first few months, no book I read helped me untangle my emotions. Friends did help, though, and over time I met other cancer-sufferers who became friends, and they helped too. My faith in God helped me put one foot in front of the other, and I found my faith growing stronger as I walked. I got across that rickety bridge, and in the years since my diagnosis I've helped others take their first step onto it.

But I've never forgotten that day in the library.

Now I've written the book I was looking for back then—a book that could have helped my brain adjust to the awful truth that I had cancer, a book that could have started me walking with confidence on the path stretching out before me.

The path may be rickety, but it is walkable. And it's possible to walk it and not stumble.

CHAPTER ONE

LOOKING AT CANCER IN A NEW WAY

Starting the journey ❧ *Good news about survival*
Giving up control ❧ *A new value to life*

CANCER CAN BE BEATEN. In fact, cancer is beaten—every day.

Going through cancer is a journey no one wants to make. It takes a lot of traveling to get back on the road to health. Who is prepared for this journey ahead of time? I'd say—no one.

Picture a woman sitting on her living-room couch. The doorbell rings. *Ding-dong.* A man stands at the door. "Congratulations," he says. "You've won a trip around the world."

"There must be some mistake," she says. "I've never even entered a contest."

"No mistake," he says, smiling as he pulls her out of her house. "You can take a plane, a boat, or a train to get you started. More than one way will get you home again, but only one way is the absolutely best route for you. You can't come back home until you've been all the way around the world. Okay? Off you go!"

"But I haven't packed."

"No time!" he calls out as she starts down the road. "Oh, and one more thing: If you don't pick the right road, your life could be in danger. Have a good trip!"

"But…" she says, looking back, "but I like it at home, and I had plans. My life wasn't supposed to go this way."

What does she do next? It depends on her personality—and what else she's already dealing with in her life.

She may be able to look ahead and start directly out on that trip around the world, thinking of all the new countries she has to pass through as exciting opportunities to experience new cultures. She may even learn a new language—or at least figure out how to say some key phrases.

She may. I know people who have taken this approach when handed the shock of a cancer diagnosis. They quickly adjust to the news, and then they're able to search out the best medical care with confidence and vigor.

I admire such people, but I'm not one of them. I am much more like the woman who, when thrust out of her house, sits down on the sidewalk with her head in her hands. *Maybe if I ignore this problem, it will go away.*

Unfortunately, cancer won't go away on its own.

I was already a doctor when I learned I had cancer, but I still needed help. Many people helped me get up off the sidewalk and start on the journey. And I appreciated my medical training. I already knew the language of medicine, and I understood its culture. Having faith in God helped, too. I knew that God loved me and that getting cancer wasn't proof that he didn't. I drew closer to him. But I still struggled to find—and then stay on—the path that would lead me back to health.

A ROUND-TRIP TICKET

I'm home again. That is, my cancer has been successfully treated. Now I want to help others who are just starting out on their cancer journeys. Each person's path will be different than mine, and I don't want to focus on my pathway as the ultimate model. So I'll share the stories of other people's journeys, also. I'm both a guide and a fellow traveler.

As a guide, I can help translate the language of medicine and explain the underlying culture. I know the route through the emotional jungle of grieving over the loss of health. I don't know the exact footpath to each person's ideal treatment, but I know the characteristics a footpath should have, and I know the warning signs that signal danger.

As a fellow traveler, I point out the family and friends who are cheering from the sidelines. I help travelers think through how God fits into their odyssey. I can comfort and encourage, and I can point toward the future as a place of hope.

SURVIVAL

When I say, "I'm home again," am I talking about "cure"? I wish cancer doctors would use the word "cure," but they won't. Unless the cancer sits entirely on some bodily surface (called cancer *in situ*) and is completely cut away, they talk about "survival" or "remission," rather than "cure."

But, you know, I can handle "survival." I like the sound of that word. I am a survivor.

Here's some good news about "survival." It's increasing. There are more than eight million Americans alive today who either have cancer or who once had it. Only 1.3 million cancers are diagnosed each year. Those numbers don't include a million additional cases of *in situ* cancers that are cured by surgery.

Doctors who treat cancer often talk about statistics. Statistics are really just a way to see the big picture, to look at trends. The trend in cancer is very good news indeed. Five-year survival rates are going up. In the 1950s only 35 percent of people with cancer lived five years or longer. By 1974 that rate had jumped to 50 percent, and as of 1997 it was 62 percent. That means 62 out of 100 people will be alive five years after they are diagnosed. Many of that "62 percent" will go on to live their expected number of years afterward, their cancer never returning. Their treatment is "successful."

Okay, doctors may not call it "cure," but the effect is the same.

And here's an even sweeter tidbit: That five-year survival rate continues to climb. America has been pouring money into cancer research for 25 years—and it has led to results. Compared to 25 years ago, treatments for dozens of different kinds of cancer are more effective and less toxic. Also, cancers are being diagnosed earlier, when any treatment has a better chance of working.

THE FACE OF CANCER IS CHANGING

Back in 1947, the outlook for people with cancer was bleak. Dr. Wendy Harpham quotes from a medical article published that year: "None of the basic problems of cancer has been solved. The death rate is constantly mounting. Small wonder that many doctors face cancer with a pessimism bordering on resignation."

Cancer treatment has made great leaps forward since those words were written. Dr. Harpham writes, "New discoveries are expanding therapeutic options every year." Medicine can do a lot to save lives, and even more to prevent suffering. Generally, far from a sense of "pessimism bordering on resignation," doctors today feel a sense of anticipation as they decide how to treat someone newly diagnosed. *I'm eager to see how this treatment will work.*

At the beginning, no one knows how a person's cancer will respond to treatment. All anyone can do is guess. However, this "guess" won't be like someone pulling a random number out of a raffle basket. It's more like guessing how many marbles are in a ten-inch jar—you can't see them all, but you can make a guess—an *educated* guess.

True, some cancers have a better chance of being success-fully treated than others do. Even though two colon cancers in two different men may look the same under the micro-scope, the first may be sensitive to a certain chemotherapy drug—that is, the cancer dies—but the second is resistant. And how the men themselves respond to chemotherapy may differ, also. One man may sail through chemotherapy just feeling a little tired, but the other man's white blood cells (which fight infection) may drop so dangerously low that he can't receive the full treatment dose of chemotherapy.

A DISRUPTED LIFE

This is no longer 1947. Treatment possibilities abound—and for every kind of cancer, there are doctors dedicated to finding even better treatments.

I know this. I knew this in 1993. So why, on the day when I was diagnosed with lymphoma, did I think I was going to die?

I wasn't responding as a doctor. I was responding as a human. "Cancer" was now a word that had been applied to me, and instantly my life had changed in a hundred ways. My mind struggled to process those changes. All of a sudden I'd become dependent and was in danger.

I was dependent, for I needed doctors to diagnose and treat me. And I was in danger, for if I didn't get treatment I'd die. And I felt wretched, which made thinking harder. When I'm sick it's hard for me to make decisions, yet here I was being forced to make decisions—*now!* I tend to panic when placed in situations like that.

And hardest of all was knowing that I wasn't in control of my life. I knew, as everyone does, that a car could hit and kill me anytime while I was just crossing the street. Life is temporary. But never had that concept seemed so real, and—if I did nothing to get treatment—so inevitable.

I hung on to God. I remember thinking about the verse from Psalm 23: "Even though I walk through the valley of the shadow of death, I will fear no evil, for you are with me." Knowing that God was walking alongside me on this journey calmed me and helped me figure out what to do.

VALUING LIFE

People who have been on a "cancer journey" are transformed in the process. We tend to see life as sweeter and appreciate it more. Not everybody diagnosed with cancer is able to get to a place where he or she is living free of cancer, of course, but everybody can be a survivor. In fact, a person with cancer is a survivor from the moment of diagnosis.

People who have never faced illness may not realize it, but life is uncertain for everyone. Each day is a gift. That's true for everyone, but cancer survivors are just more aware of it.

If you have cancer...

Consider asking yourself these questions:

- How am I responding to my cancer diagnosis at this time?

- Do I feel overwhelmed? Helpless? Or confident?

- Am I feeling hopeless or hopeful?

- Do I see myself as a survivor?

Chapter Two

Hearing—or *Not* Hearing— the Word "Cancer" for the First Time

Hearing the news ❋ *Good communication*
Being informed ❋ *Looking ahead to hope*

More than a hundred years ago Rudyard Kipling wrote *Captains Courageous,* the story of Harvey Cheyne, a teenager whose life changed abruptly. An ultrarich and pampered boy, he fell from a trans-Atlantic steamer and was picked up by a fishing vessel. There was no returning to the steamer—it was miles away by then—and the captain of the fishing vessel refused to forfeit three months of fishing to return him to port. He didn't believe Harvey could possibly be worth the millions of dollars he said he was, and besides—he needed Harvey's help with the fishing work.

So Harvey's life changed in a moment.

In the course of those three months of hard work, Harvey was transformed from a swaggering, unmanageable brat into a promising member of society. And it all started with that moment he accidentally slipped off the back of the ship.

I'd bet if Harvey Cheyne could speak with me he would be able to describe in detail his first few hours aboard the fishing vessel. He'd relate Captain Disko Troop's words: "With good luck we'll be ashore again somewheres about the first weeks of September," and how he'd protested, "But—but it's May now, and I can't stay here doing nothing just because you want to fish. I *can't*, I tell you!"

A person remembers the moments when life changes abruptly and irreversibly.

Likewise, a person who has been told, "The results of the tests show that you have cancer," is likely to remember that conversation in vivid detail—forever afterward. That was the moment when life changed.

MY MIND WENT BLANK

Most people with cancer point to the moment they were told—the moment of diagnosis—as the beginning of a new era for them. In the conversation, they remember only one statement—the first sentence containing the word "cancer." So much then swirls through their heads that they can't concentrate on the rest of the conversation.

That's what happened with Bernice B. Three days after a routine mammogram in December 2000, the technician called her and said she needed to come back in because they "had seen an abnormality."

She drove back to the hospital alone, something she regretted doing as soon as she saw the cluster of technicians surrounding the view box where her mammogram hung. She yearned for her husband to be by her side.

She wanted him even more a few minutes later when the radiologist who was on duty asked her to come to his office. "This tiny spot here could be cancer," he said, pointing to her X ray, and then he continued talking. But Bernice was no longer listening.

"I felt drained, weak," she said. "I was blinking back tears and my lips were quivering."

Before she left, a nurse made an appointment with a surgeon. "It was a week before Christmas and I remember her saying, 'Don't let it ruin your holidays.' All I could do was nod. I don't remember the doctor's name. I didn't ask him any questions because I didn't know what to ask. My mind went blank. I don't remember how I drove home."

Even though the radiologist was saying only that cancer was a possibility (though it was later confirmed), none of the words he spoke after "cancer" reached her brain.

COMMUNICATION

Communication isn't communication unless the person who is listening grasps what has been said. Doctors may tell people their diagnoses and what treatment choices they have. But if the people aren't listening, then the information isn't received—and communication hasn't happened.

At least now doctors think it's necessary to let people know they have cancer. It wasn't always so. Until the 1970s, most American doctors wouldn't tell their patients when they had cancer. Since there were few treatments, and little success with those few, doctors felt that keeping such a diagnosis secret was the only way to allow people to stay hopeful about the future.

One researcher, Dr. Donald Oken, reported in 1961 about his survey of 219 Chicago physicians. Nine out of ten favored not telling people about a cancer diagnosis, used euphemisms ("growth," "tumor," or "lesion"), and evaded further questions from their patients. "The general feeling," he wrote, "was that we can do very little to save lives and not a great deal to prevent suffering."

Even back then, Dr. Oken recognized that this situation didn't benefit people with cancer. After undergoing treatment that wasn't helping them feel better, people often dashed from physician to physician, looking for relief. A family member would be told about the diagnosis, though—and that person would feel the weight of "the awful burden of knowledge." The universal fear and dread of cancer kept people from going to their doctors if they had the slightest suspicion of such a diagnosis. This was regrettable, because even in 1961 some people were able to be cured when diagnosed early.

Dr. Oken insightfully pointed out that doctors weren't revealing the diagnoses so they wouldn't be confronted with their own unpleasant emotions. They had become doctors to help save lives, yet here they could only watch helplessly while people suffered. He urged the doctors of 1961 who were reading his article to overcome their tendency to avoid the subject of cancer, and instead to start researching ways to treat it.

NO LONGER TABOO

Medicine has come a long way since 1961. Brilliant scientists have researched different types of cancer and how to treat them. Now life-prolonging treatments are available for nearly every type of cancer. The number of people who "have had cancer in the past" is growing.

Doctors' attitudes have shifted, also. Nearly all are committed to telling their patients they have cancer. Does this mean they like to do it? No. Does this mean they are skilled at the telling? Not necessarily.

Why do some doctors have such a hard time telling people they have cancer? Because, even though a cancer diagnosis no longer means unavoidable death, it's still bad news. Sometimes very bad news.

I guess if a person was cruel and heartless, he or she could enjoy telling someone else bad news. But the vast majority of doctors are trying to *reduce* human suffering. Telling people bad news will *increase* their suffering—their emotional suffering—at least temporarily. Also, many doctors haven't faced the fact that they themselves are finite human beings with a certain number of years to live on the earth. Having a patient with a life-threatening illness makes it harder to ignore that fact.

Some doctors are very good at communicating bad news. They are more sensitive to the emotional state of their patients than others—we call that empathy. Unfortunately, the doctor-training process can be grueling, making it hard to develop empathy. Other doctors communicate bad news so rarely that when they do it they stumble over their words. Unfortunately, too few medical schools emphasize the delicate skill of effective communication.

Rejecting the Messenger

Being the bearer of bad news is tough. Back in ancient times, it was even tougher. A messenger coming to the palace from the battlefield with news of defeat might be executed on the spot. No one wanted to be the one to have to break the bad news.

Doctors aren't afraid of execution when they tell people they have cancer, but they may be afraid of the emotions that result. People's disappointment at such a diagnosis may turn into anger—anger directed against the bearer of the bad news.

An article in the *British Medical Journal* states, "The worst fear for doctors—particularly junior doctors—is that the patient will blame them personally for the bad news that they bring." As doctors become more experienced, they learn to recognize this as a natural human reaction and understand that they are not the true target. This emotion may be natural, but it's still unpleasant to be the object of such anger.

"We're seldom angry about what we think we're angry about," wisely writes Cecil Murphey in *Simply Living*, a book that expands on the meaning of various biblical proverbs. The proverb he was reflecting on was "A soft answer turns away wrath, but a harsh word stirs up anger." By answering "softly," a wise person can help the angry person see what the root of the anger really is—a feeling of injustice, perhaps, or of life not going as expected, or of fear.

Too few doctors know how to give a "soft answer" in the face of anger. Those who do are usually more willing to give bad news when it's needed, for their patients' anger doesn't "stick" when it's directed at them.

FACING FEELINGS

Doctors are people. Just as people have different personalities, life experiences, and goals, so do doctors. Some doctors avoid the emotional aspects of their patients' lives, seeing medicine as purely a science without emotional involvement. I think this was a more common perspective a generation ago, when science was making so many breakthroughs. Many illnesses were being understood and successfully treated for the first time in history. Medicine seemed crisp, neat, and readily explainable. Why focus on something so unpredictable as a person's inner reaction?

In 1980 Dr. Franz Ingelfinger urged doctors to reconsider their approach. He was the well-respected editor of the *New England Journal of Medicine* when, three years before he died of stomach cancer, he gave a now-famous speech in which he urged doctors to change. They should avoid medical terms that "laymen either do not understand or misinterpret" and sensitize themselves to their patients' emotions. "Distraught by anxiety, fear, and perhaps suspicion, the patient hears the sound but not the meaning of words."

How people first hear they have cancer impacts their health—both emotional and physical. One research study found that women who thought their physicians lacked empathy when they told them they had breast cancer had a harder time coping with the necessary treatment.

When people don't know the facts, they're likely to use their imagination to fill in the gaps. And that tends to be far worse than the truth. "Not knowing about one's clinical reality is often associated with uncertainty and unrealistic fears, a condition that patients describe as 'worse than knowing the facts.' Becoming well-informed may enable patients to maintain hope by freeing them from anxiety and fear."

THERE'S A REAL BENEFIT IN BEING INFORMED

Doctors often view cancer from a different angle than their patients do. Cancer is conquerable. Doctors know there are many treatments "out there," whether or not they know what they are. The average person, though, thinks cancer means inevitable, sudden, and painful death—or worse, a lingering and agony-filled death. Even though the road ahead is a challenge, what a doctor has to say today is full of hope. As one doctor wrote,

> Clinicians often are concerned that providing patients with detailed information about their disease may create despair. It is useful to know that helping patients become well-informed does not create depression but actually assists many patients in sustaining hopeful attitudes.

The key word is hope. People who are hopeful handle the bumpy road ahead better and are happier with the life they are living as they are going through treatment. It doesn't have to be a hope for cure, or even for remission. Hoping for freedom from pain, for growth as a person, and for quality time with family members may be just as satisfying as hoping to live to reach 90.

THE BEST WAY TO BE TOLD

So how should people be told they have cancer? In studies and surveys, researchers have learned how people want to be told:

- face-to-face by their own doctor, a doctor with whom they've had some prior connection

- in an ideal world, with a cancer specialist in the room also—one who is available to answer questions about the path ahead

- in a room separated from the hustle and bustle of the office

- without interruption by cell-phone calls or pagers

Sometimes people want a family member or close friend in the room with them, and sometimes they don't. Almost never do they want other medical staff members there, even if they are kindhearted people.

And what about the words the doctor uses? What is the best way for a doctor to break the news?

- gently, yet with "we'll-put-up-a-good-fight" attitude

- with all of the medical information that's available, but no bleak statistics

- with assurances they'll be pointed toward effective medical treatment and if it proves to be ineffective there will be other options; also, that any of their pain will be dealt with, and that they won't be abandoned

And people might not want to hear everything at one time. In other words, people want the truth—but with compassion.

HOPE LOOKS AHEAD

So how often does this happen? How often do people first learn of their cancer in a private, quiet room in which their doctor, with whom they already have a relationship, has asked an oncologist to be present also—and both doctors are sensitive, caring people who also have a good understanding of what treatments are available and how to access them?

I would guess...never.

Does anything in life ever happen in the most perfect way? No, and yet we learn to live with it. More than 500 years ago Thomas à Kempis wrote, "Be not angry that you cannot make others as you wish them to be, since you cannot make yourself as you wish to be."

So even if a person was told in the worst imaginable way—in a rushed and impersonal setting by an uncaring and distracted messenger—it's still possible for that person to choose to go forward.

Hope looks ahead. Anger looks behind.

RELEASING THE PAIN

To go forward, though, a person may first need to turn back briefly—in order to forgive. If a woman, for instance, feels deeply wounded by the way a doctor told her she had cancer, then she has a choice on how she will respond. She can let that pain fester, or she can release the pain by forgiving the person who has hurt her.

"Someone once said that staying angry is like taking poison and waiting for the other person to die," wrote Frederica Mathewes-Green. By choosing to forgive—and spitting out the poison—a person lays the groundwork that will allow healing to take place.

If you have cancer...

Consider asking yourself these questions:

- How did I feel when I was first told I had cancer? Have my feelings changed since then? If so, how?

- Is there anything about the circumstances under which I was told I had cancer that is keeping me from moving forward? If so, how can I resolve those issues so that I can look ahead toward healing and health?

- Do I need to forgive someone who has hurt me?

CHAPTER THREE

ADJUSTING EMOTIONALLY TO THE DIAGNOSIS

Everything changes ❋ *A new reputation*
Grief ❋ *Dealing with emotions*

I CAN RELATE TO BILBO BAGGINS. He is the "hobbit" in J.R.R. Tolkien's book of the same name. On the day the story opens, Bilbo is living a peaceful, orderly, and comfort-filled life. He stands by his door after breakfast, minding his own business—as hobbits generally do.

Then Gandalf, the powerful wizard, appears.

"Gandalf came by," Tolkien wrote. A simple statement, yet for Bilbo Baggins it meant that his life had veered off in a radically new direction.

Gandalf invites Bilbo to participate in an adventure, and although Bilbo resists ("Sorry! I don't want any adventures, thank you. Not today. Good morning! But please come to tea—any time you like! Come tomorrow! Goodbye!"), two days later he sets off on the dangerous quest that fills the rest of the book.

Bilbo Baggins, by nature, desired a calm, structured life. I'm not a hobbit, but like a hobbit I'm fond of making plans and then generally expecting them to work out. When cancer entered my life, I wanted to say, "Sorry! I don't want it, thank you. Not today. Good morning! Goodbye!"

But cancer came—uninvited—and swept me off onto its own timetable for a year.

THE MOMENT WHEN EVERYTHING CHANGED

In April 1993 I was a part-time physician and a more-than-full-time mom. I had a two-year-old daughter and a one-year-old son, and was 15 weeks into a pregnancy that had left me weak and nauseated from the day I found out I was expecting. The evening hours were the worst.

So on the evening of April 6, Don, my kind husband, was tubbing the kids so I could collapse on our blue recliner. I brushed my hand against the left side of my neck.

That's odd, I thought. *What are these lumps?*

I examined myself. Hard, painless lumps—a mass of lymph nodes stretching from my earlobe to my collar bone. I forced my brain to think about what they might mean. Only one word formed—*cancer.*

What kind of cancer could it be? Lymph nodes are the "sewage-treatment plants" of the body, the place where germs get killed after draining out of nearby body parts. Cancer also drains into lymph nodes, and you can figure out which organ has cancer by observing which lymph node is swollen.

So where's the cancer that's causing these lymph nodes to swell? I asked myself. Everything I could think of—cancers of the head and neck—needed massive surgery and serious treatment.

Out of the tub, Martha Grace zipped past me, squealing as Don came running after her. Pete was in his arms, wrapped in a towel. He squirmed to the floor, and now Don was chasing both of them, all three laughing. The moment—so familiar, for it was a bath-time tradition—now struck me as immensely precious. The scene hung in my memory, and indeed it hangs there still.

It was the moment when everything changed. There was the "before"—the 34 years when I didn't have cancer—and the "after." I had just entered my "after."

The doctor part of me was sure I had cancer, although I didn't know what kind yet. But the human part of me didn't believe it at all. *I couldn't have cancer.* It seemed hazy and unreal.

After the kids were asleep, I asked Don—who is also a doctor—to examine the lymph nodes on my neck. Before touching them he said breezily, "I'm sure they're nothing." His attitude reassured me, even though I knew he was wrong.

After touching them, though, he frowned. "Now I'm worried," he said. I didn't want to hear that. My chest tightened, and I felt like I was smothering.

We didn't sleep much that night. I kept waking up and thinking about the baby growing inside me. *Does my having cancer put this precious life at risk? But maybe I don't have cancer.*

The Balloon Slips out of My Grasp

It was as if I'd just let the string to a balloon marked "health" slip out of my hand, and now—despite my lunging after it—the balloon had floated upwards and was drifting farther away. I wanted time to go backwards. *Next time, I'd keep a tighter grasp on that string.*

But the balloon was out of my reach. Within two days I had a lymph-node biopsy that confirmed my fear. I had cancer.

Don was the one to tell me. My surgeon had told him while I was still groggy from anesthesia, so when I woke up he was sitting by my bed.

"Is it cancer?" I asked him.

He nodded, taking my hand. I couldn't breathe. "It's Hodgkin's lymphoma," he added.

"Hodgkin's?" The stifling heaviness lifted, and I could breathe again. "That's treatable, even curable." I felt relief and dread all at the same time. For two minutes Don and I just looked at each other, our hands clasped.

Then my questions tumbled out. *But what will happen to our baby? Where should I go to get treated? And what about the plans I already have for next week? Next month?* I didn't want to have cancer. I didn't want to be sick. I didn't want my life to be disrupted—but I was beginning to realize it already was.

A DARK REPUTATION

I wonder if there's ever been anyone who has stayed calm when cancer has entered. "Thank you, doctor, for letting me know I have cancer. Now, how are we going to treat it?" That's no one *I've* ever met.

I ask this because I have taken care of people who have calmly accepted other diagnoses—even though they were just as life-threatening, or even more so. Heart failure is one such diagnosis—three out of four people with severe heart failure will be dead within five years. Yet I can't convince some people that they are in serious danger and need to stop smoking (if they smoke) and take their medicine.

So why is cancer so alarming? After all, it's a treatable disease. The treatment process is tough to endure, but it's not always painful. Even cancers that can't be cured can often be beaten back again and again—a process that sometimes goes on for decades. Lots of living is still possible.

I think the word "cancer" has so much emotional overlay for people because for centuries it meant certain death. The light of today's promising treatments has to penetrate centuries of dark reputation.

Another emotional blow people have to deal with is having to change the way they see themselves. I know this was true for me. I found myself being forced to acknowledge, "I am someone who has cancer." Accepting this reality faced me with a shift inside my brain. I didn't want it to be true, but at the same time I knew it *was* true. I wanted to stay in the past and not step into the present.

I had started to grieve.

❧ UNDERSTANDING GRIEF ❧

What is grief? Grief is a response to loss. It's the way we respond to the loss of something or someone important to us. Grief is a process. When the loss is great, getting to the place of acceptance takes time and work—*grief work.*

Calling it "work" is appropriate, for it is, indeed, *work* to get past all the powerful feelings that bubble up when we experience loss. No two people follow the exact same path through grief, yet there are enough similarities in everyone's experiences so we can talk about "the stages of grief."

STAGE ONE: SHOCK AND DENIAL

In the "shock and denial stage," the loss seems unreal—like the haze of a bad dream. The mind is unwilling to accept the reality of the loss. That's what my mind was doing when I first knew I had cancer. I was holding back the flood of pain that would come when I accepted that I had, indeed, lost my health—even if only temporarily.

I'd lost something else, too. I'd been thinking that I had life under control, that I was in charge of what happened to me. That turned out to be an illusion, an illusion that was now shattered.

I stayed in this stage for several days. I looked normal on the outside, I was able to talk appropriately about having cancer, but my whole self wasn't really engaged in these conversations.

Four evenings after I had first felt the lymph nodes on my neck, Don and I went out to dinner to celebrate our eleventh anniversary. Don is not an emotionally expressive person—I've rarely seen him cry. Yet he reached for my hand and said, through tears, "I'm not ready to give you up yet."

"Thank you," I said, "I'm not ready to go, either." But I was thinking, *What a sweet thing to say, and look how touched he is.* I remember feeling detached from the scene—like an outsider looking in. Don was clearly feeling an aching sadness, but I felt like I was in a Plexiglas cube, protected from his world of pain.

STAGE TWO: EXPRESSING EMOTIONS

All that changed the next day. I was keeping a journal, and my journal entries for the first four days had recorded events—many facts and few feelings. But on the fifth day I poured out a flood of fear and uncertainty.

I had shifted into the second stage of grief, "expressing emotions." The doorway to emotional pain had appeared before me, and to move forward I needed to open the door and step through the doorway. What about other emotions that might flood me if I let this fear in? What would I do with anger *(This is not the way my life is supposed to go),* despair *(I'm going to die),* and guilt *(Surely I caused this cancer by something I did)?*

By refusing to open the door I'd avoid the pain—at least for a while. But that would mean I'd stay in that first stage of grief, a state of fuzzy unreality.

I know people who have refused to step through that doorway. In medical terms it's called "denial." This is, for instance, the woman who refuses to believe that the lump in her breast might be anything other than an infection—and no, she doesn't want it removed. It is the man who insists God has healed him of lung cancer, although the chest X ray still shows the ugly spot. It is the woman who skips follow-up appointments for her leukemia, telling the receptionist who calls to check on her that she's feeling fine right now and has some important things to attend to and will be in next week.

Precious days, weeks, and sometimes months go by—time that could have been spent diagnosing and treating a cancer that was still in its early stages, when the chance of cure was greatest.

Stepping Through the Doorway

In his classic book *Good Grief,* written to help people make sense of what they are going through, Granger Westberg wrote,

> God has so made us that we can somehow bear pain and sorrow and even tragedy. However, when the sorrow is overwhelming, we are sometimes temporarily anesthetized in response to a tragic experience. We are grateful for this temporary anesthesia, for it keeps us from having to face grim reality all at once....Shock is a temporary escape from reality. As long as it is temporary, it is good. But if a person should prefer to remain in this dream-world rather than face the reality of his loss, obviously it would be very unhealthy.

People whose brains are numb shouldn't make important decisions. If they do, they're likely to be unhappy with the outcomes further on.

Here's the hard part—the early weeks of a cancer diagnosis are peppered with the need to make one crucial decision after another. People who are floating in a state where everything seems unreal can't focus on all the facts. Only if people are willing to step through the doorway into the painful stage of "expressing emotions" can they get to the place where they can make careful, reasoned decisions that will benefit them.

Hitting the Ground Hard

I jumped out of an airplane once. Just before my college graduation I signed up for a one-day lesson in parachuting, which ended with a jump. Over and over the instructor told me to check my main parachute as soon as I was out of the plane to see if it had opened automatically as it was supposed to. If it wasn't open, I'd hit the ground in 17 seconds—unless I pulled the cord on the backup parachute.

As the plane climbed to 3000 feet I reviewed my instructions: *Jump, arch back, check for open parachute.* No problem.

Then I jumped—but not only did I fail to arch my back (they told me later I scrunched myself up like a ball), but I didn't check my parachute until halfway through the three-minute jump. The sensation of floating and the beauty of the scenery had mesmerized me. If the first parachute hadn't opened on its own, I'd have hit the ground long before I'd had the presence of mind to open the second one.

For the first few days after I learned I had cancer, I was floating. I couldn't have made a reasonable decision—or pulled an emergency-parachute cord—during that time.

Happily, I didn't need to. Even though my cancer was growing rapidly, I had a few weeks to get plugged into a course of therapy before I'd be in great danger, as most newly diagnosed people do. Also, I had a husband who loved me and was thinking clearly—well, at least a lot more clearly than I was. He helped so much with those early treatment decisions.

After those first few days, the ground rushed up at me and I hit earth with a thud. That is, I started to experience emotional turmoil. Trivial events triggered tears. When people helped me care for my children—and I needed their help—I anguished over the thought that I wasn't needed anymore. Would I ever be able to function on my own again? I was angry that I couldn't plan ahead, for cancer is the ultimate "schedule disrupter." My emotions tumbled and surged.

I could have begged for drugs—prescription medicine that would deaden the emotional pain—but I didn't. I knew that taking them would slow my adjustment to this new reality. Instead, I cried out to God for help. I particularly remember reading the Psalms at this time. David, who wrote many of them, spoke to God with blunt honesty. And he asked God the questions I'd been having trouble putting into words:

> O LORD, hear me as I pray; pay attention to my
> groaning. Listen to my cry for help, my King and
> my God, for I will never pray to anyone but you.
>
> I cried out to you, O LORD. I begged the Lord
> for mercy, saying, "What will you gain if I die, if
> I sink down into the grave? Can my dust praise
> you from the grave? Can it tell the world of your
> faithfulness? Hear me, LORD, and have mercy on
> me. Help me, O LORD."

David is saying, "Keep me alive so I can still praise you!"
I like that. I feel a strong kinship with David.

Numbing the Pain

Many people do ask for—and get—prescriptions for
drugs that lessen anxiety. Or they use alcohol, for which they
don't need a prescription, to smother their anxiety. They are
distressed, after all, and they want relief. But anxiety is an
expected step in the grieving process of people who have just
found out they have cancer.

As a doctor, though, I know how inviting it seems to "just
write a prescription." I ache inside when I see people suffering from emotional pain. They want relief. I want them to
be relieved. Didn't I choose medicine as a career to help relieve
human suffering? My hand reaches for my prescription pad.

But if people are suffering because they've just been told
they have cancer, numbing their emotions wouldn't be truly
helping them. I have to remind myself that the pain they're
feeling is temporary and that suppressing it won't make it
evaporate. The anguish of their new diagnosis will still be
there—under the surface—and will need to be dealt with
eventually. When the pills are gone, it'll return, and then it
may be bigger, uglier, and harder to work through.

Besides, people who have just found out they have cancer
need every bit of their capacity to think clearly. If their brains
are fuzzy, they'll tend to make decisions they'll later regret.

I wish people could put off making any major decisions until they are completely through with this stage of grief. People in emotional turmoil have a hard time evaluating which options before them are best. Dr. Jimmie Holland, who has worked with thousands of distressed cancer patients at Memorial Sloan–Kettering Cancer Center in New York, describes this in the book *The Human Side of Cancer* (co-written with Sheldon Lewis). She notes how hard it is (though necessary) to make decisions at this time when "fears are exaggerated far beyond the actual likelihood of their happening."

> It is important to realize that this turmoil is a common, normal response to the threat to your life. You are not "going crazy." It is unfortunate that important decisions about treatment must be made during this time of high distress when thinking clearly is apt to be most difficult. Today, many people seek several opinions about what the best treatment might be, and the opinions are often different.

Moving Forward

So what does "expressing emotions" look like? Does it mean we can dump our ice-water buckets of emotions on our friends anytime we want to? Do we now have permission to scream at our children and say hateful things to our spouses? Am I encouraging people to be like the woman who—while waiting ahead of me in the supermarket checkout line one day—turned and told me everything she was angry and resentful about?

No. Actually, I'm trying to keep people from becoming her.

I suspect that woman had had a terrible loss at one time in her life, and she had plunged into grief. She got to the "expressing emotions" stage, but then became stuck. She either refused to move on, or she couldn't, without help—and none was available. And now everyone she encounters gets a piece of her anguish.

This second stage of grief should be temporary—a "temporary turmoil." It may look like a woman allowing herself to cry when sadness overcomes her, or a man admitting to his wife that he's scared. Life has become different, and our emotions need some time to catch up to that fact. Some of those emotions need to be expressed—at the right time and in an appropriate way. How they are expressed will be different for every person.

Tears Are Okay

When I'm grieving, not everyone I know will be supportive. Some people can't handle another person's expressing emotion. It reminds me of the time I was talking to a woman who had just heard me speak on the process of grief.

"Thank you for putting into words exactly what I've been going through," she said. "My neighbor died just two days ago and I'm having a really hard time."

"How tough that must be for you," I said. "Was she a good friend?"

As she nodded, her eyes filled up with tears. I grabbed her hand and squeezed it. Just then, another woman, who seemed to know the first woman and who had been waiting to talk with me, interrupted.

"You'll be okay," she said to the woman firmly. "Just trust in God." The woman nodded, pulled her hand away from me, and blinked back her tears. She had gotten the message—emotions are not allowed.

I tried to say something that would give her permission to express her pain, but she shook her head, smiled, and walked away. Did crying over her friend's death mean she wasn't trusting God? Of course not.

When we express our pain, we need to choose our "listeners" wisely. Usually people have someone in their lives with whom they can talk on a deep level—the level where emotions are shared. If not, or if those people seem more hurtful than helpful, there are counselors available to be that "listening ear."

Sometimes, too, a "new loss" will uncover an "old loss" that was never dealt with. In that case, a counselor may be needed to help a person work through the grieving process, since the emotions of the "old grief" are still under the surface. Those emotions are no longer fresh—they've been allowed to fester—and handling them is beyond the person's strength.

There's nothing shameful about getting counseling help when it's needed. A counselor can give insight into and perspective on what seems to be an unmanageable situation.

STAGE THREE: ACCEPTANCE

So what's the goal—and the benefit—of plugging away at this painful process of grief? It is getting to a place of "acceptance," the third stage of grief. If the emotions have been dealt with in the second stage, they won't be as strong now.

Granger Westberg calls this final stage of grief "affirming reality." There is a new reality—an unpleasant, unwanted reality—and we're beginning to figure out how to live with it. He writes,

> We finally begin to affirm reality. Please note that we do not say that the final stage is, "We become our old selves again." When we go through any significant grief experience we come out of it as different people.

After a significant loss, life will never be the same. People don't forget the way it used to be, and they may very well wish it was that way again. "Accepting" doesn't mean "forgetting."

If I'm chopping carrots and my knife slips and gashes my hand, I will have an open wound. It'll hurt. I'll try to protect it so it won't get infected—for infection would keep it from healing—and slowly it will scab over, and eventually it will become a scar. I'll always be able to point to the place of the gash because I'll see the scar. But scars don't hurt.

Likewise, when I've come through grief I can remember my loss, and point to it, but I no longer feel a surge of emotions. The wound has healed.

In normal grieving, people who have reached this final stage of grief are beginning to see the whole picture. They're gaining a perspective on how this loss fits into the rest of their lives. They are making plans for the future—plans that acknowledge that what is lost is, indeed, lost.

It usually takes several months to reach this stage of grief. After all, the process of getting cancer diagnosed and treated comes with a swirl of uncertainty that keeps churning up emotions. *Will my cancer respond to treatment? Will I reach remission? Will I need to change treatments in a few months?* No one knows.

The upheaval of the second stage of grief distracts me and drains my energy. The sooner I can accept this new and unpleasant reality of cancer, the sooner I can fight it with all of my strength.

In my case, I was also dealing with the "hormonal surges" of pregnancy. Every mother wonders whether the baby inside her will be safe and will be born healthy. I just had a lot more reason to wonder.

After five months of chemotherapy, I went into labor, and John Newton Givler was born. He came five weeks earlier than his due date, but he was fine. Really fine. God had kept him safe.

In the last chapter of *The Hobbit,* Gandalf accompanies Bilbo back to his home after a year's absence. It was a year filled with harrowing adventures. Just before they arrive home, Bilbo pauses to recite a poem about traveling and then returning. Gandalf recognizes that this is a new Bilbo. Through the struggles of the journey, his companion has grown and developed. "My dear Bilbo!" the wizard says. "Something is the matter with you! You are not the hobbit that you were."

If you have cancer...

Consider asking yourself these questions:

- ❧ People who are grieving commonly pass through similar "stages":

  shock and denial

  expressing emotions (fear, sadness, anger, despair, guilt)

  acceptance

  How would I describe right now my response to the diagnosis of cancer?

- ❧ Have I begun to "affirm reality" by accepting that my life has changed?

CHAPTER FOUR

ENTERING THE MEDICAL WORLD

A new experience ❧ *Understanding "distance"*
The need for a doctor ❧ *Looking for compassion*

IN THE FIRST STAR WARS MOVIE that came out ("Episode IV"), young Luke Skywalker joins up with the wise old Obi-Wan Kenobi on a mission to fight the evil Empire. Just before they enter a bar in the big city where they hope to hire a spaceship and pilot for their journey, Obi-Wan warns Luke, "Watch your step. This place can be a little rough."

But Luke is cocky. "I'm ready for anything," he replies.

A minute later Luke is standing at the door, gaping at dozens of bizarre aliens, all of whom are drinking and talking. The camera zooms in on his face as he scans the smoky bar. There's an alien with a head like a hammerhead shark, and the musicians playing snappy jazz music have huge hairless foreheads. A creature that looks like a snake is talking to a fuzzy wolf with menacing teeth.

And there Luke stands at the entrance. He's trying to look comfortable, as if he's familiar with this kind of place, but his wide eyes betray him. Clearly the "anything" he was ready for didn't include *this*.

Entering the System

When I watch that scene, I remind myself that at least Luke Skywalker *wanted* to be there. That bar was the first step of an adventure he was excited about being on. He got himself together pretty quickly. By the time he found Obi-Wan at the back of the bar, he no longer appeared ruffled.

I wonder how long it would take Luke to adjust to the setting of a modern hospital. He enters a hospital hallway, and people—all purposeful and in a hurry—stride past him. But who is who? That bearded guy in the blue scrubs—is he an emergency-room nurse, a surgeon, or an aide from the orthopedic floor? And that woman in the white coat—does she draw blood in the lab, or is she a staff psychiatrist?

"Excuse me. Move aside," a young man calls, pushing with one hand a white-haired woman seated in a wheelchair, and with the other a rattling metal pole with swinging bags of clear liquid.

I suspect that Luke would be uncomfortable—and that his discomfort would last longer than it did when he entered that smoky bar. And that's assuming he's completely healthy.

But what if he'd recently been told he had cancer and had come to the hospital for vital treatment? He wouldn't want to be there—or, rather, he wouldn't want to *have* to be there. His anxiety and dread would interfere with his ability to take in the new sights, sounds, and smells.

Getting Around in a Foreign Country

To have cancer means treatment. And treatment means doctor's offices, radiology departments, hospitals, and—often—large medical centers.

In a medical building, the walls are bright, the floors gleam, and—though this is less true now than it used to be—the defining color is white. It's enough to disorient anyone, especially someone who doesn't know which shimmering hallway is the right one.

But just as Luke Skywalker eventually became comfortable dealing with aliens, people with cancer eventually learn how to navigate medical centers. In *The Complete Cancer Survival Guide,* Peter Teeley writes about his experience of getting his colon cancer treated at Georgetown University Medical Center's Lombardi Cancer Center:

> Setting foot in the Pasquerilla Healthcare Center on my way to the Lombardi wing was like entering a Metrorail subway station at rush hour, with people bustling to and fro. By my third visit, though, I felt completely at home.

It's hard for doctors to realize how foreign a hospital can seem to someone who is not used to it. And many doctors come from medical families and so have walked hospital hallways since childhood. For them, it's even harder to imagine feeling ill at ease in such a setting.

A visit to even a doctor's office can be intimidating. The new patient passes through a packed waiting room—past a droning television—to reach a large sliding window, behind which sits the receptionist.

ADAPTING TO REALITY

I certainly remember when I was first learning my way around a hospital, which was during my third year of medical school. By the time I was diagnosed with cancer, I'd spent 13 years roaming the halls of hospitals. It felt strange to be a "receiver" of medical care rather than a "supplier," but the setting itself didn't bother me. It was my world.

So because I was already comfortable, I knew some things about hospitals and doctors that helped me get better care—or at the very least, more pleasantly given care. For instance, I knew better than to harshly insist on my own way, to repeatedly ask the receptionist when my name was going to be called, or to spend my entire clinic visit complaining about my aches and pains.

But what am I saying? Wasn't I the one who was hurting, the one dealing with the emotional blow of having cancer? Weren't medical people there to help me, and wasn't it their job to do so compassionately? Yes, in an ideal world. But I don't live in an ideal world. I live in a world filled with people whose computer crashed last night, or whose alarm clock didn't go off when it was supposed to this morning, or whose daughter has had a nasty cough for a week. I live in a world filled with humans, each of whom has human weaknesses. Their being able to get through the training to become a doctor, a nurse, or an X-ray technician didn't change that fact.

I also live in a world filled with people who don't want to die. They don't want to die, and yet the knowledge that they will—someday—lurks deep in the back of their minds. More than any other serious illness, cancer—or meeting someone with cancer—seems to drag this awareness out into the open and bring uneasiness.

FEELING A GROWING DISTANCE

Alice Stewart Trillin, though not a doctor, was invited to write an essay about her experiences as a cancer patient for the prestigious *New England Journal of Medicine*. She wrote, "Our fear of death makes it essential to maintain a distance between ourselves and anyone who is threatened by death." She had felt some of that "distancing" from her friends when she was first diagnosed with cancer. That saddened her, but didn't surprise her. But she also felt it with her doctors, and that did surprise her. She observed, "If we get well, we help our doctors succeed; if we are sick, we have failed." She suspected that her doctors feared death.

True, doctors—taken as a whole—have met more people with cancer than has the rest of the population, but they still are surprisingly unlikely to have faced—and accepted—the reality that life on earth has an end. I believe the same is probably true for other clinic and hospital employees.

So, as I worked my way through the medical system as a patient, I tried to stay aware that I would make many people uncomfortable just because of my diagnosis. I'd try to expect little from the people caring for me when I first met them, and I would work to make a personal connection over time. I tried to remember that some of them were ecstatic over being there at work, but that many others were counting the hours until Friday—or the days until retirement.

If I was treated rudely by someone, I gave that person the benefit of the doubt. (Okay, okay—I *tried* to give that person the benefit of the doubt. I did not always succeed.) Maybe he was just having a bad day. Maybe she had run out of gas on the way to work that morning.

As Philo of Alexandria said long ago, "Be kind, for everyone you meet is fighting a great battle."

Joy in a Dark Place

I think Philo of Alexandria would have liked one of my patients, whose first name is—appropriately—Joy. The way she lives her life illustrates his quote. Joy D. is someone who, despite suffering with pain, cheers up the gloomy person beside her in the waiting room—and cheers up the whole waiting room at the same time. She reminds me of Paul and Silas, whose story is told in the Bible. The book of Acts reports that they were put in prison for telling people about Jesus in the early years of the Christian church. They were singing—singing!—while sitting shackled in prison after having been attacked by a crowd and then stripped and flogged by the town leaders.

Joy had been my patient for several years when, in 1999, she came to me with a stomach pain that kept getting worse despite the several medicines I prescribed. I knew something was wrong, and she did, too. I ordered medical tests, but they all came back "normal." Her pain increased. But instead of becoming irritable, she became even more upbeat and positive.

"I know you'll figure out what's wrong, Dr. Givler," she told me more than once. "It's just a matter of time."

What effect did this have on me? I yearned to help her. I intensely wanted to find out what was wrong. I remember that, on the days when I'd seen her, I would spend all the time of my drive home thinking through the possibilities of what could be causing her pain. I'd still be thinking about her the next day. When she was finally found to have large-cell lymphoma, I don't know which of the two of us was more relieved to finally have a diagnosis.

But how I wished that diagnosis hadn't been cancer! She was stunned, too, but soon her hope returned. "There could have been another bad thing wrong with me that would have been worse than the cancer," she said, "something not as treatable. I was glad that since I did have a cancer, it was a treatable one."

Joy's words amazed me. How could she respond that way? I think that some of that optimism came from her basic personality—and that a big boost came from her faith. "I believe in God," Joy said. "I know he'll help me." Her outlook helped her get through a medical system that can seem uncaring and neglectful—without ending up angry and resentful because of the way she'd been treated.

"I knew God was using those people to help me," she told me recently. "I thought it was important to be cooperative with them. I know how easy it is to get aggravated with a nurse, or a doctor, or an aide. I just took that to the Lord: 'Lord, help Dr. So-and-So. He's needing you right now.' I called that 'turning it over to the Lord.' Then I needed to leave it there."

TIRED BODY, COLD HEART

The process of becoming a doctor is often such torment that compassion is simply squeezed out of a person. More than once during a night without sleep while I was a resident, I remember asking myself, *Why should I be nice to this patient* (or this family member, or this nurse) *when I'm so drained and so stressed?* I behaved—frankly—like a jerk.

I felt sorry for myself and thought I had a right to be cranky. I'm not proud of those memories. Today, after the benefit of many good nights of sleep, I deeply regret many of the interactions I had with people while I was a resident.

After I finished my residency, I consciously decided to never again work that many hours a week (often more than a hundred). Such stress will almost certainly take a toll on a person's outlook on life. In an article on doctor–patient communication in the *British Medical Journal,* the authors write, "Medical education is a stressful and sometimes abrasive experience that can produce cynicism and callousness."

Surely every doctor practicing today started out as a first-year medical student who thought compassion was important and who planned to make every interaction with a patient pleasant. For some, though, that priority got buried under the avalanche of medical knowledge they were expected to absorb. A hundred years ago the brilliant Sir William Osler said, "To cover the vast field of medicine in four years is an impossible task." And that was a hundred years ago! Medical knowledge has exploded since then.

NARROWING THE FOCUS

Early in the twentieth century, doctors realized they couldn't learn all there was to know about every part of the body. And so, many doctors began to "specialize" in certain organ systems in order to more fully grasp everything there was to know about that area.

As a family practitioner, I know "a little about a lot." Specialists know "a lot about a little." I thank God for specialists. I have needed specialists' expertise many times and have benefited from their knowledge. But it's very hard—maybe impossible—to focus on one part of the body and still keep in mind all the other parts.

And then there's something even more elusive—seeing the big picture, the person as a whole. I remember being taught in my family-practice training to think about how a person's illness fits into the context of the rest of life. How does being sick impact the person's emotional well-being? And what is happening to the person's family?

I know many specialists manage to keep this in mind, too, which is all the more admirable because I doubt it was emphasized in their training.

Sir William Osler was famous for his teaching ability. His students (medical students and young doctors) loved him. But his patients loved him too. They knew he was thinking about them as human beings. "Care more particularly for the individual patient," he said, "than for the special features of the disease."

WHAT YOU NEED IS A DOCTOR

In the same speech in which he urged doctors to be sensitive to their patients' emotions, especially when telling them bad news, Dr. Franz Ingelfinger also told of being diagnosed himself—with stomach cancer. The standard treatment was surgery—which he underwent—but what further treatment he needed wasn't clear. Radiation therapy? Chemotherapy? Both? He reported, "At that point I received from physician friends throughout the country a barrage of well-intentioned but contradictory advice."

He became "increasingly confused and emotionally distraught." Finally a wise physician friend told him, "What you need is a doctor." What his friend meant was that he needed someone to assume responsibility for his care. He took his friend's advice, and he and his family "sensed immediate and immense relief." He finally had a doctor who was thinking of him as an intact person, with an emotional self that was connected to his physical self. His emotions had swelled within him and were overpowering him—he was no longer able to make careful, reasonable medical decisions.

Unfortunately, many people who are diagnosed with a serious illness nowadays don't have such a doctor coordinating their medical care. Maybe they'd never before established a relationship with any doctor because they'd never needed one. Or maybe they'd had doctors, but never one who had looked beyond their unwell bodies to see how they were thinking and feeling.

Later in his speech, Dr. Ingelfinger calls the tendency of doctors to ignore the emotional state of their patients "a lack of empathy."

> Doctors for various reasons find it difficult to put themselves in the patient's place; they do not sufficiently appreciate, or perhaps do not have the time to appreciate, how the patient feels and how he reacts to the medical information and procedures to which he is exposed.

He refers to not having the time for empathy, and I think this is increasingly the case. Most doctors are under tremendous pressure to see too many patients in too little time. Many doctors schedule so many patients per hour that they couldn't possibly have an in-depth conversation with each one.

ABSORBING THE SHOCK

But I think there's another force at work in addition to time pressure, and that is doctors' need to protect their emotional selves. All doctors put some emotional distance—a "buffer"—between themselves and their patients. This is healthy for doctors (for they'd soon get swallowed up by their patients' collective distress if they didn't), but it also benefits their patients. Without a tangle of emotions to work through, doctors can more effectively apply their medical knowledge to the situation at hand.

Cancer doctors care for people with complicated medical needs. Because so many of their patients are seriously ill, I suspect they have an even greater emotional buffer than do other physicians.

Doctors can have a buffer and still have compassion. And I highly prize the compassionate touch. I want it for myself when I am a patient. When I am going to see a doctor I don't yet know, I ask people who know her, "What is she like as a person?" Long before my first appointment I'll try to find out how she treats patients.

If my problem is complicated, I'm willing—for the sake of seeing someone with specialized knowledge or skill—to sacrifice this desire. But given a choice between two competent doctors, I will choose the more compassionate one every time.

When I was diagnosed with cancer I entered the world of medicine as a patient. Though it was a familiar world to me—no Luke Skywalker there, and no aliens—it unexpectedly felt strange and different as I experienced it from a patient's perspective. Learning my way around it helped me get the medical care I needed. It can be done.

Those who walked that way before me helped me see where to go. I stood on the shoulders, so to speak, of those who were treated before me. And those treated after me will be able to see even farther because they'll be standing on mine.

If you have cancer...

Consider asking yourself these questions:

- How do doctors' offices and hospitals make me feel?

- Do I have a "doctor"—someone whom I can trust to assume responsibility for my care? If not, can I find one?

- As I walk through the health-care system as a patient, do I try to remember that receptionists, technicians, nurses, and doctors are all people, with many of the same stresses and pressures that I face? Do I try to accept their shortcomings in the same way I would like them to accept mine?

CHAPTER FIVE

HOW MEDICAL CARE
BECOMES TRUSTWORTHY

The importance of observation ❧ *Testing brings reliability*
Good research leads to good medicine ❧ *The personal touch*

I AM GLAD I WASN'T PREGNANT in Vienna in 1844. That's the year Ignaz Semmelweiss started working as a doctor at the Vienna Lying-In Hospital, where the women of the city went to have their babies.

But I would have been happy to meet Semmelweiss. He was apparently a sensitive and compassionate doctor. What I'd want to avoid was the hospital itself.

The hospital was split into two sections—the First Hospital, where medical students trained, and the Second Hospital, where midwives trained. Women begged to give birth in the Second Hospital. For in the First Hospital, childbed fever raged—with a death rate of up to 30 percent. In the Second Hospital, the death rate was only three percent.

Semmelweiss grieved at the deaths of all these young mothers while the other doctors "shrugged their shoulders. They called the disease an epidemic, perhaps due to overcrowding, nervous tension, or cosmic influences. Such deaths had been happening for many years. It must be the way things were meant to be."

No one understood about germs.

Semmelweiss struggled to find the answer to these tragic deaths. Why the difference between the two hospitals? He spent much time in the autopsy room attached to the First Hospital, as did all of the medical students. The midwife students weren't allowed in the autopsy room.

Finally his eyes were opened. The culprit was Semmelweiss himself—and the medical students. They would leave the autopsy room—where they dissected the dead bodies of women who had died of childbed fever—and go directly to the bedside, where they did internal exams of women in labor, perhaps rinsing their hands a bit beforehand. With horror Semmelweiss realized that he himself had infected many women with childbed fever.

He began insisting that everyone leaving the autopsy room wash their hands thoroughly with a mild bleach solution. The death rate plummeted—down to one percent.

First Observe, Then Check It Out

Semmelweiss was a scientist at a time most doctors weren't. That is, he used the scientific method: See a problem, figure out a possible solution, and then test to see if that solution "works." He saw suffering that didn't make sense, and so he struggled to figure out why. He stayed alert for clues. He observed. Then he saw a possible explanation. He checked it out and found that it was, indeed, the reason for the suffering.

Just suggesting a possible explanation isn't enough. It must be "checked out"—that is, tested. This step is what separates so much of the health advice given by well-meaning people who are concerned about a particular form of suffering from the health advice given by the traditional medical community.

That process of "testing" is *research,* and it's what—ideally—traditional medicine is based on. So if I eat a litchi nut when I have a stomachache and—voilà!—the stomachache vanishes, I haven't proved anything. Even if I give a litchi nut to my husband who also has a stomachache and thus cure him, I still haven't proved anything. To prove that litchi nuts cure stomachaches, I'd need to do a research study with two groups of people: one that is eating litchi nuts and one that is eating a nut that looks like a litchi nut but isn't. Then I'd compare the results from the two groups.

THE BIRTH OF MODERN MEDICINE

After uncovering the cause of childbed fever, Semmelweiss spent the rest of his life—18 years—trying to convince other doctors of the benefits of cleanliness. Tragically, he was only slightly successful. Doctors weren't used to practicing medicine differently based on the results of carefully documented research.

Happily, now they are. The era of "modern medicine," which I define as medical practices based on clear evidence that they are helpful, began with a French doctor, Pierre Charles Alexandre Louis. Dr. Louis lived at the same time as Semmelweiss, and he studied a medical practice that hadn't been questioned in thousands of years—bloodletting.

To say that bloodletting was deeply rooted in medicine is an understatement. Hippocrates describes it as a standard treatment for several diseases—especially infections—and that was 500 years before the birth of Jesus.

Back when George Washington developed a serious throat infection in 1799, his doctors suggested bloodletting, and he readily agreed. I think they went a little overboard, though, even by the standards of the day. It sounds like they removed at least six pints of blood—maybe more—over half of his total supply. He died within 24 hours.

What Dr. Louis did was compare two groups of people with lung infections, for which the standard treatment of the day was bloodletting. One group underwent bloodletting during the first four days of illness, and the second group underwent it later. The first group had more deaths.

I think even Dr. Louis was surprised. No one had questioned bloodletting before. After that study, doctors began to look for evidence that a particular treatment would be beneficial before they gave it.

THE TESTING PROCESS

Why is testing various treatments important? Because this is what makes medicine reliable. Medical care is more than just one person's idea of what seems to be a good thing to do.

To the extent that a treatment has been tested, to that extent it's applicable to other people who need it. Sometimes people with cancer are going to be asked to be part of the testing process. But far more often they will be the ones to benefit from the experience of other people who have been part of the testing process before them. The testing process is the key.

So much is not known about cancer. But so much *is* known, too. It's known because researchers have been studying different cancers—and how they respond to various treatments—for decades. But there is still much to learn. For anyone part of the process, knowing the way research is done, and the terms researchers use, is essential.

Modern medicine is forward-looking. The general attitude is not "We already know everything about this disease," but rather "As much as we know—and it's a lot—we're sure there's an enormous amount we don't yet know." So in every area of medicine there are researchers who are studying how people respond to new treatments. Maybe these treatments will turn out to be better than the established ones.

RESEARCHING RESEARCH

Some people have even done research on how to do research! The best studies, they've found, have five key features: They are *prospective, randomized, placebo-controlled, double-blind,* and *statistically significant.*

Researchers have learned that asking people about their past—how much exercise they've gotten in the last year, for instance, or what their diet has been like for the past five years—is not nearly as accurate as gathering a group of people and then seeing how much exercise they really do, or what they're actually eating. These are *prospective* studies, and they have been found to be more valid than *retrospective* ones.

Researchers have also learned that if people think they are getting a medicine that will help them—to relieve pain, for example—one out of three will be helped regardless of what the medicine is. In fact, it could be a sugar pill. They call this the *placebo effect.*

The Worthy Placebo

Some people sneer at the placebo effect, but I don't. If I'm not sure whether a medicine will relieve someone's pain, I don't say, "There's only a slight possibility this will help." No, I say, "I think this will help you." I want my patients to get better. Why not boost their chance of healing by a third?

I apply this to myself, too. I don't like to hurt. So, when I take aspirin for a headache I say to myself, "The moment I swallow this the pain will disappear," even though, deep down, I know aspirin doesn't take effect for 30 minutes. But often the headache is gone—instantly. I love the placebo effect. I want it on my side.

Before a new medicine can be sold, researchers have to find out whether it's effective. So they gather a group of people who have the disease the drug is supposed to treat and divide the group in two. Actually, a computer divides the group—randomly. Thus the study is *randomized.*

Half the original group receives the new medicine, and the other half, a placebo. If a third of the people in the group that get the medicine improves, but so does a third of the placebo group, then the drug isn't effective.

These days nobody gets a placebo without being informed and giving consent to the possibility. Also, if there's already an effective medicine for a disease but researchers want to see if a new one is even better, they give the established medicine to half the group, and the new one to the other half. The group of people who get the established medicine is called the *control group*. If they get a placebo instead, then the study is *placebo-controlled*.

Avoiding Bias

Researchers have learned that everyone can be biased. If the doctors giving the medicine don't believe it will help (because, for instance, they know it's just a sugar pill), they will unintentionally convey their doubts to the people receiving it. Or they may want the new medicine to work so much that they deem the people who received it as more improved than they really are. So researchers ensure that not only are the people taking the pills ignorant of which group they're in, but so are the doctors who give the drugs and evaluate how well they're working. The doctors are "blind," and the patients are "blind," so the study is *double-blind*.

Finally, researchers have to study a large enough group of people. If they don't, then the results they get might have come about by chance alone. Usually this means at least 30 people in the group that gets the new treatment and 30 in the control group. The more people they can study, the more likely the study will be *statistically significant*.

Just discovering that a new treatment is effective isn't enough. What will it do to advance the world of medicine if only a small group of researchers know about a great new therapy? They now need to try to publish their results in a medical journal so that doctors everywhere can learn about the new treatment. In their published paper they also describe exactly how they did the study—and the closer they've stayed to the "prospective, randomized, placebo-controlled, double-blind" ideal, the fewer critics they'll have. Their study may be so convincing that the new treatment becomes the standard way to treat that illness.

RECEIVING QUALITY CARE

Some illnesses have a standard way to treat them—children with diabetes need insulin, for instance, and people without a functioning thyroid gland need a pill to replace that hormone. But most illnesses are treated in a variety of ways. Cancer, taken as a whole, is like that.

Rarely do all oncologists agree on one single way to treat a certain cancer. Many cancers have national guidelines for treatment, though, and most oncologists treat the more common cancers in ways that are close to these guidelines. Because two cancers that look the same under the microscope can behave very differently from each other, treating cancer can get very complicated very quickly.

Sometimes what is considered standard care in one part of the world, or in one part of the country, is markedly different from that in another part. Doctors are generally aware of their locality's standard. If they vary their treatment too far from that standard and a particular patient doesn't do well, that patient may end up suing them for malpractice. Not every doctor has been sued for malpractice, but every doctor dreads the possibility. Being sued is a bulldozer that flattens a doctor's confidence.

A group of Wisconsin researchers who studied the effect of malpractice suits on the doctor-patient relationship concluded,

> The litigation experience and the perceived threat of litigation encourage patients and physicians to view one another not as partners in a health care program, but as potential adversaries

in multi-million dollar lawsuits. To begin a therapeutic relationship on the basis of suspicion makes
conflict—legal or otherwise—virtually inevitable.

Too many malpractice suits stem from a breakdown of
communication between the doctor and patient. The patient
didn't feel the doctor's compassion. And ironically, the very
thought that he or she might get sued may make a doctor
fear and distrust a patient. And a swirling attitude of fear
and distrust strains communication.

Alternative Medicine: Alternative to What?

People want their doctors to be compassionate and
caring. This builds their trust, and trust is key in the
doctor–patient relationship. When people don't trust their
doctors, they're likely to seek care somewhere else. And in
the case of "alternative medicine," that is exactly what has
happened.

What exactly is alternative medicine? It's not just one
thing. When people turn from traditional medicine and seek
an alternative, they embrace a diverse group of treatments
and philosophies.

I think there's a common thread, though. Those who
practice alternative medicine listen to the people who come
to them, and they spend time with them. They have a personal touch. Also, most of them tend to see a person as a
balance of the physical, mental, and spiritual selves. This
appeals to everyone who is convinced people have a deeper
dimension beyond just their bodies.

When Dr. Wendy Harpham was diagnosed with an
incurable non-Hodgkin's lymphoma, she chose to be treated
by an oncologist, but was surprised at the number of
people who suggested alternative treatment. "Family,
friends, and strangers bombarded me with stories, information, and advice about diet, doctors, the mind-body connection, and alternative treatments." She filed all that

advice away while she received "conventional" treatment. After a year's remission, the cancer came back, and that's when she opened up those files to see what alternative medicine could offer.

> The lure of alternative therapy was powerful but I knew that not all hope is equal. Realistic hope—hope based on fact—is stronger than that born of wishful thinking, which is why my desire for a sense of control over my disease was overshadowed by my resolve to learn the facts about my treatment options and base my decision on them.

In her probing of alternative therapies, what Dr. Harpham found was a lack of scientific studies. There were many personal stories of recovery, but maybe those people would have gotten better anyway. The studies that conventional medical care is based on—the *prospective, randomized, placebo-controlled, double-blind,* and *statistically significant* studies—were nonexistent.

Of course, carrying out such studies takes time, and people with cancer feel a sense of urgency because their lives are in danger. But many herbal treatments are now being studied in a scientific way, and some look promising. They may be part of "conventional medicine" soon. After all, powder from the bark of the willow tree was first used in standard medicine in 1763, but it was a folk medicine long before that. Today we know it as aspirin.

Some forms of alternative medicine may never be studied in a scientific way because they're founded on a philosophy that clashes with science. A book put out by the Center for Bioethics and Human Dignity states, "Many forms of alternative medicine claim that physical healing is based on the manipulation of a nonphysical human energy field, one that cannot be detected by physical instruments." Since such a "human energy field" cannot be detected, it can't be measured. This makes studying it difficult.

HIGH-TOUCH AND HIGH-TECH

The best medical care is based on solid scientific evidence—evidence for the fact that it has a good chance of helping—yet is still given with a personal touch. People who are physically hurting are looking for support, comfort, and hope. Drawing from her 25 years of experience, Dr. Jimmie Holland writes, "Reflecting on my work with people with cancer, I have come to the view that the more high-tech the treatment a patient must go through, such as bone marrow transplantation or repeated cycles of high-dose chemotherapy, the greater the need for 'high touch,' since the emotional and human needs are greater."

The best medical care is like the ball used in the game of baseball. No one can play baseball with a billiard ball—too solid. Nor a tennis ball—too hollow and bouncy. But a baseball has a solid core (of cork and rubber) and a soft leather cover. Caring for people should be based on a core of solid scientific evidence, but have an outer, visible layer that is understanding and supple.

If you have cancer...

Consider asking yourself these questions:

- How confident am I in the ability of standard medical care to treat my cancer? How do I feel about "alternative medicine"? How will I decide whether to choose one form of treatment or the other, or even both?

- How much do I want to know about the scientific basis for the treatment that I am receiving? Am I comfortable following my doctor's recommendations, or do I want to do research myself so that I better understand the available treatments?

CHAPTER SIX

CHOOSING A HEALTHY ATTITUDE

Harmony in one's life ❧ *Thinking about the future*
Good attitudes toward treatment ❧ *Finding hope*

THE STORY OF CHARLOTTE AND WILBUR is one of the greatest
love stories in all of literature. True, it's not "love" in the
romantic sense, but it's the love of a friendship in which each
member sacrifices for the other—and considers doing so a
privilege. The fact that Charlotte is a spider, and Wilbur a
pig, doesn't diminish the beauty of their relationship.

As a child I loved E.B. White's *Charlotte's Web*. I
remember anticipating the day I'd be introducing its magic to
my own children. Back then I little thought it would still cap-
tivate me also. But each time I've read it out loud to our children—as I've neared the end, and Charlotte dies—I have
sobbed.

A spider's natural life span is a fraction of that of a pig.
Charlotte knew that. Wilbur didn't. So Wilbur didn't know
what he was asking when he pleaded with an aging Charlotte
to come with him to the county fair. She had written words
in her web that described Wilbur's finer features, and this
had made him famous. Then she came to the fair and spun
another word, "humble," which clinched his fame and won
him a special award. Now he would not be butchered. She
had saved him.

But her own life was coming to an end. "Why did you do all this for me?" Wilbur asked her.

"You have been my friend," Charlotte answered. "That in itself is a tremendous thing. I wove my webs for you because I liked you."

Charlotte knew what she wanted to spend her life on, and her resolve didn't waver even when she knew her days were few. I've always suspected that the energy she spent on weaving webs with words shortened her life. She didn't dwell on that possibility, though. She used her last strength to give of herself to the pig that she loved.

THE BIG PICTURE

I admire Charlotte—and I'm a little in awe of her. When I am suffering, I tend to think only of my own comfort and my own needs. But she seemed to see so clearly how her life fit into the "big picture" of life on earth, and she understood that Wilbur was worthy of her help.

Her outward focus reminds me of the story of Stephen from the book of Acts in the Bible. The religious leaders didn't like what he was saying—in fact, they didn't like it so much that they stoned him. Being hit with rocks must have been agony. Yet just before he died, he cried out, "Lord, do not hold this sin against them." So even in his moment of extreme pain and peril, he prayed that God would extend mercy to those who were killing him.

This amount of selflessness jolts me.

The ancient philosopher Epictetus wrote, "It is difficulties that show what men are." That quote makes me think of an elderly man—a retired minister—who was my patient when I was still in training. He had diabetes and required insulin shots to lower the sugar level in his blood. In the few, soft words he spoke he usually managed to squeeze in a reference to his love for Jesus. I also noticed that he treated his wife, who always accompanied him, with kindness and respect.

One day, as soon as I arrived at the clinic I heard a commotion. Someone was yelling at full volume in the room where the nurses check people's blood pressure. I rushed back there and found my elderly patient thrashing his arms and legs wildly as he sat in the chair. "Thank you, Jesus!" he bellowed. "I love you, Lord! Yes, God, yes, Lord. Praise you, Jesus!"

I quickly learned from his wife that he'd been sick to his stomach that morning, and so he hadn't eaten anything. But he'd still taken his insulin. His blood sugar was dangerously low, and all that he'd just said hadn't been under his control. We got some sugar into him, and soon I had a mild-mannered gentleman before me again.

He was unaware of what he'd said a few minutes earlier, and when I told him, he was embarrassed.

"But I don't think you should be embarrassed," I said. "Quite the opposite. I admire you because I see a lot of integrity in your walk with God."

"Why is that?" he asked.

"Because when you were not in control of yourself, then who you really are—deep within—came out. And who you are on the inside harmonizes with who you are on the outside." His wife was nodding. She did not seem surprised.

I haven't seen this man in years, but I think about him a lot. I want to be like him—the "inner me" in harmony with the "outer me."

INVESTING IN THE FUTURE

Sometimes cancer has already spread extensively by the time it has been diagnosed, and so has little chance of being eliminated. With such a diagnosis, some people plunge into despair, whereas others remain confident, maybe even cheerful. Why the divergence? And does the course people take make a difference in the outcome of their illness?

In April 1993, a week before I was diagnosed, another young family doctor in our community was also diagnosed with cancer. In fact, David C. and I were the same age and had trained together. With a loving wife, a son, and two daughters (the youngest three years old), he wanted to live. But the forecast for his particular cancer was nothing like mine. He had renal-cell cancer, which had already spread beyond the kidney at the time it was diagnosed. Because of how aggressive a cancer it was and how poorly this kind of cancer tended to respond to treatment, his doctors told him he had only a 10-percent chance of living five more years. With the treatments commonly available at the time, he'd probably only live six to twelve months.

Because I was fighting my own battle for life, I had only marginal contact with David for the first ten months of his treatment, but after that we talked frequently. I remember one conversation we had after he'd just learned that his cancer had spread further despite the treatment he'd been getting. His statistical chance of surviving five years had now dropped to 5 percent.

"I'm not thinking about the 95 percent," he said. "Why can't I be one of the 5 percent who survive?"

Why not indeed? Someone had to be in that 5 percent. Why not David?

David researched his treatment options and found some doctors at a hospital in Los Angeles who were doing innovative renal-cell cancer treatment, with promising results. He spent two weeks out there initially, and then made many more trips for further treatment and follow-up. His cancer shrank at first, but then it began spreading again, so he researched and found other therapies that looked hopeful. He chose to aggressively pursue treatment. It was a big investment.

But his investment paid off. He lived four years after his diagnosis, 36 more months than anyone had offered him hope for. Those were months filled with time with his children—giving input, helping them with schoolwork, making memories. He wrote his children letters that described his hopes for each of their lives. He organized his finances and made sure his wife knew where all the important papers were. His relationship with God became stronger and more meaningful. And in a letter to his friends that was read at his funeral he wrote,

> *The thought of leaving [my family] without a husband and father, imperfect as I am, has been the hardest thing for me to deal with. I think this thought has helped me to hang on as long as I have. For the past four years, through 6 operations, through 3 rounds of radiation therapy, through all the medicine and chemotherapy, the thought of my wife and children has strengthened my will to continue fighting and trying to get well.*

For four years David's goal had been clear: to regain his physical health. He fought to get well again. That goal didn't keep him from considering the needs of the people he could still influence. And that goal didn't keep him from doing things that would benefit his family if he did die. But we who knew him agree: David had a fighting spirit.

Do I Need a Fighting Spirit?

I heard a lot about "fighting spirit" when I first got cancer—that having an "I can conquer this" approach toward cancer would help beat it back, and I wondered whether there was scientific evidence that supported this idea.

In 1979 a British researcher named Dr. Steven Greer, along with two colleagues, published the results they'd obtained by following 57 early-breast-cancer patients for five years. The women had all received a simple mastectomy as their only treatment (appropriate at that time because of the early stage of their cancers). Dr. Greer had categorized the women into four groups depending on how they were coping with their illness. The categories were

* *denial*—active rejection of any evidence of their diagnosis (10 patients)

* *fighting spirit*—highly optimistic, looking for information, determined to fight the cancer (10 patients)

* *stoic acceptance*—cancer is acknowledged but they don't seek out information unless new symptoms develop (32 patients)

* *helplessness/hopelessness*—overwhelmed by diagnosis and lives disrupted by preoccupation (5 patients)

Dr. Greer's results suggested that the women who coped with *denial* or *fighting spirit* had a greater chance of remaining alive than those who coped with *stoic acceptance* or *helplessness/hopelessness*. In a later study, Dr. Greer added another category, *anxious preoccupation,* which was defined as persistent anxiety about the diagnosis and a tendency to interpret every piece of information negatively. Women in this category were also less likely to survive five years than the women coping through denial or fighting spirit.

This study was the beginning of a flood of controversy. Some people grabbed hold of this study and concluded that everyone with cancer had to mentally fight their diagnosis with a frontal attack, or else they would surely die—and if they did die it would be their own fault. But this study wasn't asking—or answering—that question. Others pointed out that the number of women followed was too few to make broad, sweeping conclusions. Because of the few women followed, Dr. Greer himself urged people not to generalize on the basis of his study alone. Also, the study began before doctors understood the importance of lymph-node involvement—which now they know to be crucial—in assessing the risk of dying of breast cancer.

Many follow-up studies have been done. Dr. Jimmie Holland, who has spent her career helping people cope with cancer and has published many articles on the subject, has written,

> Over the years, many studies have been conducted to clarify the role of personality in health. The studies have frequently found contradictory or inconclusive results. This is largely because of the difficulty in carefully studying psychological and physical domains at the same time.

In other words, some studies show a connection between a person's approach to coping and length of life after diagnosis, and some show no connection. All studies have focused on one particular cancer or another—breast cancer and melanoma have been the most frequently studied—so no study has tried to encompass all types of cancer.

The Burden of Guilt

One large study by Dr. Maggie Watson and her colleagues followed 578 women with early-stage breast cancer for five years. Here the research didn't confirm the earlier study by Dr. Greer. Women with the "fighting spirit" mind-set did not have improved relapse-free survival compared to those with other mind-sets. The researchers concluded, "Our findings suggest that women can be relieved of the burden of guilt that occurs when they find it difficult to maintain a fighting spirit."

The burden of guilt. I certainly experienced the burden of guilt. I remember one time when a friend called, a few days after I'd gotten a dose of chemotherapy.

"How are you doing?" she asked.

"I feel pretty wretched," I said. I knew my voice was flat—I certainly felt that way.

"You've got to perk yourself up, Amy," she said. "You've got to apply your mind to fight that cancer."

"Right now I don't feel like fighting anything. I'm just lying here in bed trying to endure."

"No, Amy. You've got to think *positively* or it might not go away."

I remember hanging up, my insides churning as I unsuccessfully tried to convince myself she was wrong. I didn't have any energy to fight, so if she was right—and the cancer didn't go into remission—my lack of positive thoughts would have caused it.

Now that I have looked at the medical research, I realize that my friend's advice came from a misinterpretation of what has been studied—a misinterpretation I've since heard many times from other sources. I've found no research proving a clear-cut link between a "fighting spirit" coping style and a better treatment outcome.

FINDING HELP AND FEELING HOPEFUL

But I can see how another coping style—"denial"—could definitely affect outcomes. That is, if people so completely deny their cancer that they don't seek out treatment, or if they miss appointments and ignore worrisome symptoms because they don't really believe they have cancer at all, then their survival will obviously be affected. "Complete denial" is one way of coping, but it is not a healthy one if it paralyzes a person when action is necessary.

Dr. Maggie Watson's study did show that those people whose mind-set was "helplessness/hopelessness" when their cancer was first diagnosed were less likely to survive than people with the other mind-sets. She suggests one reason this might be true: People who hold a helpless mind-set don't seek out the amount of health care needed to maximize their chance of survival.

Surely someone who is crushed at the thought of having cancer and thinks *I'm going to die and nothing anyone can do will help,* will be less likely to follow up with needed medical treatment, as well as less likely to eat a healthy diet, get some exercise, and seek social support.

In other words, people who are feeling helpless seldom seek out help, and people who are feeling hopeless have given up on the future.

Similarly, it makes good sense that people whose basic coping style is "fighting spirit" will keep all their appointments, will ask their doctors questions, will make sure they understand how to handle problems, and will search for cutting-edge treatments. If cancer researchers have recently had a breakthrough in treating a certain cancer, then people with "fighting spirits" are more likely than anyone else to find out about it and then travel to get that treatment before their local oncologists are routinely giving it.

But people with "stoic acceptance" mind-sets can function well also. They might not ask a lot of questions, but they're probably doing fine if they stick with their therapy, eat a basically healthy diet, and seek out the emotional support they need. They don't need to be forced into a mental approach that doesn't fit their personalities.

There Is Always Hope

Hope is vital. Hope is necessary even when a cancer has already spread before the time of diagnosis—as it had in my friend David C.'s case—and there is little chance of cure. Dr. Holland writes,

> The opposite of hope, hopelessness, is a devastating emotion that saps the psyche in a profound way. It takes away energy, purpose, and the

strength to interact with others at a time when this is so important....There is always hope, even when it is grounded in stark reality.

David showed me he had a fighting spirit by his drive to get the most promising treatments—but at the same time he was realistic. When I spoke with him over the years, he would acknowledge the small—and shrinking—possibility his cancer could be removed. Yet he didn't give in to despair. He realized he had a choice on how to live each day, even as he seized every chance to add to his days. He was outward-focused, thinking of the future, even if that future might not include him.

SLOW AND STEADY

Many times through the four years during which I followed David's pursuit of effective treatment, I remember wondering whether I would have—or could have—kept going as long as he had. Could I have mustered that much energy? I know he viewed his strength as coming from God, so maybe God would give me the same strength in the same situation. Still, I admired his pursuit of life.

When I consider the four approaches to their cancer that Dr. Greer saw in the women he studied, I think I fit more in the "stoic acceptance" group rather than the "fighting spirit" one. (Or how about "stoic acceptance with a bit of hysteria and panic thrown in"?) The language commonly used in cancer literature is the language of war: fight, battle, combat, destroy. These words don't resonate with me. I want my cancer to be gone, but I'm happy for it to just slip away from my body—and the more gently it can be removed, the better.

Dr. Greer's definition of "stoic acceptance" includes "not seeking further information," and that does not characterize me. I did seek further information, and I wanted to understand the reasoning behind every medical decision.

But during my months of treatment I did not wake up in the morning thinking, *Today I'm going to jump up and conquer this cancer!*

I think I'm more like the tortoise in Aesop's fable "The Tortoise and the Hare," plodding along to get the task done. By simply continuing forward, eventually I crossed the finish line.

POSITIVE THOUGHTS

I'm now thinking of another friend of mine, whom I'll call Heidi. If anyone could have been said to have a fighting spirit, it was Heidi. We met when I was finishing up my chemotherapy and she was just starting. I liked her instantly. We both had three young children—and we both wanted to be around to raise them.

Heidi had a lymphoma—like I did—but hers was resistant to the first chemotherapy her doctors tried. She then found out what various lymphoma experts around the U.S. were doing for her type of cancer, and she flew across the country to get treatment advice from several of them. She bought hundreds—maybe thousands—of dollars worth of vitamins and herbs. Never did she acknowledge to me that there was any outcome possible other than complete cure. She spoke only positive words. I suspect she thought only positive thoughts.

She came home from one trip saying that the doctors had declared her to be "cancer-free." She died two months later.

Apparently people closer to Heidi than I was had an inkling that the doctors really hadn't declared her to be cancer-free. They urged her to make audiotapes of advice for her children as they grew. They urged her to write down her impressions of her children so they could have them later on. Even if she lived, that effort wouldn't have been wasted. But she refused, insisting such things weren't needed.

A week before she died it was obvious to everyone—even her—that she was dying, but by then she didn't have the mental stamina to record a message or write anything down. I don't know if she had even made a will. I hope she did.

Maybe if Heidi had allowed herself to squarely face the possibility of death, she would have crumbled emotionally—for a time. I'm sure it would have been a painful process, but I think she eventually would have gotten past it. Then she could have given her husband a chance to prepare too—and they could have walked the last leg of her journey hand in hand.

Heidi's story still makes me sad—and maybe my emotions are too tangled up in it for me to be objective. But part of my entanglement comes from seeing myself in her story. I wonder whether I would do the very same thing, were I in her situation. In my grasp for more life, what would I miss in the lives of my loved ones? I don't want to forget that the way I face the future affects more than just me. I don't want to miss the big picture.

A TRULY HEALTHY ATTITUDE

The most provable type of research has a clearly defined endpoint. For instance, "Taking aspirin right after a heart attack will save the lives of one out of every forty people who do so." Such research asks the question, "What is the end result—life or death?" The answer can be measured—it's crisp and exact.

So I can understand why the cancer researchers studying the difference between various mental outlooks chose to look at "time to death" or "time to first relapse" as the endpoints. The answer can be reported with precision. But there are other measurements of successful treatment that are more elusive—and just as important.

For example, did having cancer awaken a certain woman to what was really important in life, and did she then pursue that thing? Or, even though this man's body wasn't healed, was having cancer the spark that encouraged him to work to heal damaged relationships? Was she able to forgive and receive forgiveness? Did he spend his available energy and time focusing on his family members and their long-term needs? Did she grow closer to God?

Perhaps having responses such as these doesn't extend life. Nobody knows—no studies have been done. Maybe life isn't longer, but surely it's fuller. If I were doing a study on mental attitude in cancer, I think I'd try to study these types of responses. But I don't even know how I'd begin to measure them. Maybe they're simply not "measurable."

I guess the measurement would have to include additional people, not just the person with cancer—and that would get complicated. After all, do any of us really know the impact we are making on others?

The writer of the book of Acts reports that, when Stephen was stoned to death, "the witnesses laid their clothes at the feet of a young man named Saul." Saul's name was later changed to Paul, and he helped spread Christianity, but at the time of Stephen's stoning he was trying to kill off Christians. Did Stephen's selfless response to his own death influence Saul? Many Bible scholars, beginning with Augustine in the fourth century, believe that it did. Augustine declared, "The Church owes Paul to the prayer of Stephen." And how many people have been impacted by Stephen's life—and death—by reading about him in the book of Acts?

In *Charlotte's Web*, Charlotte may not have known the impact she was having on Wilbur, but her example stayed with him the rest of his life. Charlotte's example deeply affected Wilbur, and it has affected me, too. I am inspired by the way Charlotte—and the biblical Stephen, and my friend David— chose to relate to other people. They each left a legacy behind.

If you have cancer...

Consider asking yourself these questions:

- How am I coping with my diagnosis?

    denial?

    fighting spirit?

    stoic acceptance?

    anxious preoccupation?

    helplessness/hopelessness?

    How is this affecting the way that I approach my medical care, my daily life, and my relationships with my family and friends?

- What reasons do I have to be hopeful for the future?

- What is the "big picture" in my life? How has having cancer changed my understanding of what is really important? What can I do to make my life fuller and more productive? How can I positively influence those around me?

CHAPTER SEVEN

THINKING THROUGH THE OPTIONS PROMPTLY

Taking action • *Getting a second opinion*
Evaluating providers • *Considering fertility issues*

THOUSANDS OF PEOPLE WERE INSIDE the two World Trade Center towers when first one, and then the other, were hit by airplanes flown by terrorists on September 11, 2001. Those inside One World Trade Center had 100 minutes between the moment of impact and the collapse of the building. Those inside Two World Trade Center had less than an hour.

Of course, no one knew the buildings would collapse. No one knew they must not only get out of the buildings, but far away—blocks and blocks away.

Instant decision-making and quick action were called for—and in many cases they determined people's survival.

Yin Liang, working on Lehman Brothers' e-commerce Web site on the fortieth floor of One World Trade Center, had sat down at his work station only 20 minutes before the time when—at 8:48 A.M.—he heard a rumbling boom. Then the entire room started swaying—first one way, and then the other. He stood up and—along with a dozen co-workers peering over their cubicle walls—looked out the window. Dark chunks of debris were falling past them.

"What happened?" someone called out.

Yin felt his chest constrict. Something was deadly wrong. But nothing within the room had changed. He stood there, forcing his mind to think as he watched through the window.

Then a member of another team strode past him, heading for the emergency exit. Seeing him shook Yin awake. He followed immediately—without even picking up his bag.

"Let's go!" he called out to his teammates, who were still standing, looking startled.

"But what's going on? What happened?"

"Get out of the building *now!*" he and others shouted back. One senior manager, Tom Kruger, poked his head in every room to make sure all employees had gotten the message—especially those in inner, windowless offices. Eventually, everyone made it off the floor.

Once out of the building, Yin kept walking. Not until he was two blocks away did he turn and look up. He stood frozen. Dense smoke poured from the tops of the towers. Others around him stared upward—some from as close as a block away—but Yin knew this was not the time to pause. He had long admired the ancient samurai warriors of Japan, and knew he must continue to act decisively—like a samurai. So he kept walking north, and was far from the towers when they collapsed.

Yin Liang's day had veered off in a radically unexpected direction, but he was adjusting to the changes—and was willing to take action even though he didn't fully understand all that was happening.

People diagnosed with cancer need those same qualities:

* forcing the mind to think
* making decisions promptly
* acting on those decisions
* keeping focused on the path ahead
* staying alert to the possibility of change

Having them could lengthen their lives.

GOOD CELLS GONE BAD

Thinking about how my cancer originally formed shocks me a bit. At some time in the past, one little lymph cell, snug in a lymph node, lost all its inhibition. It started multiplying, and soon there were thousands, then millions, of wild little lymph cells. They weren't listening to the rest of my body. Nor were they doing what lymph cells were supposed to be doing—helping my immune system function. No, these little lymph cells were not looking out for the good of the total organism—me. Instead, they were intent on only one thing—making more copies of themselves.

My own body had gone haywire, or at least a bunch of my own cells had. I felt betrayed. Every minute that went by meant that more of these crazy little cells were in existence. They had to be stopped. I'm sure my own immune system was trying to snuff them out, but it wasn't keeping up with their growth. The firm, matted lymph nodes on the side of my neck that had first alerted me to my cancer grew larger by the day.

I could hardly blame my own immune system, though. It was designed to destroy foreign invaders, and here were cells—its own cells—that looked very similar to healthy cells. Could I expect it to perceive that they were, in fact, enemies?

My immune system needed some help, and from the day I was diagnosed, I was actively seeking that help. I didn't know what form the help would come in—would it be surgery to learn the full extent of the cancer? chemotherapy? radiation?—so I was looking for people who had enough knowledge to make that decision.

Who to go to? The choices seemed endless.

Right away I knew I wanted to go to a doctor who specialized in cancer—an oncologist. In my residency training I had worked in a cancer clinic, and—though I had tried to absorb what was going on—I had come away from those four weeks having learned just one big lesson: Treating cancer is complex. Cancer is not, after all, a single disease.

There are more than a hundred different cancers, each with reams of information available about it—who is at risk for getting it, what it acts like, and how it's treated. There are experts on each separate kind of cancer who have devoted their careers to it.

Information Overload

Most cancer doctors treat a wide range of cancers. This usually means that, over time, they become most comfortable treating the cancers they see more often—the common ones. They are most likely to stay up-to-date with the treatments for those cancers. No one can know everything there is to know about every kind of cancer. The field is just too huge.

And even if it were possible to be so incredibly brilliant as to be able to learn everything about—say—ten different cancers, and to have an amazing memory that retained all that information, within six months a good chunk of that knowledge would be outdated and no longer useful. That's because cancer researchers are constantly studying new treatments, comparing them with the old, and publishing the results as journal articles.

I just did a search on *PubMed,* an Internet site for medical articles that is made available by the National Library of Medicine. It has short descriptions of all the articles in thousands of medical journals published worldwide. I searched for the word "cancer" in articles published in the last six months. There were more than 18,000 such articles on that subject. Then I limited my search to just the "core clinical journals." Those are the hundred-or-so journals with good reputations that target doctors who are treating people (that is, not primarily doing research). A still overwhelming 2784 articles popped up. Anyone who took the time to read all of those articles—or even to skim them—wouldn't have time to take care of patients.

It takes a lot of time to take good care of cancer patients. And not every "cancer doctor" is actually taking care of patients—at least, solely taking care of patients. Many do research, which takes a lot of time also. This is more true at the major cancer centers scattered throughout the country.

Doctors who want to really immerse themselves in information about a particular type of cancer, and who want to be around others similarly interested, tend to gravitate to these major cancer centers. Often they must do research as a condition of their employment, but this is what most of them want to do anyway. Being in an environment where research is encouraged may be the main reason they are there. They may teach in a nearby medical school also, and may travel frequently to teach other doctors. All this takes time.

So what happens when someone wants to go to a major cancer center? Let's say a woman has just been diagnosed with multiple myeloma. She wants the most up-to-date treatment available. She learns about a "Dr. Wowser," one of the world's foremost authorities on multiple myeloma. She makes an appointment, then travels several states away to the major cancer center where he works. Her actual time with that doctor may be brief. If she receives her treatment there, other doctors may actually take care of her in the hospital. She may become part of a "clinical trial" that is investigating a promising new treatment. Or she may not stay at the cancer center. After getting Dr. Wowser's advice on what is the best treatment for her, she might then travel home to have her local cancer doctor administer it.

SECOND OPINION

Getting that expert doctor's advice is called "getting a second opinion." Doctors at major cancer centers are often asked to give a second opinion, which almost always means the person with cancer travels to see the doctor, usually bringing the pathology slides that show the cancer cells. That way, the doctor—or, more likely, the pathologist at the center—can look at the slides and make sure the diagnosis is correct. Often, the person with cancer gets a few more X rays or other tests at the cancer center.

A second opinion is routine. Doctors aren't shocked when a patient asks for one, and most of them welcome the influx of new ideas. Dr. Jimmie Holland, who works at Memorial Sloan–Kettering Cancer Center, where thousands of second opinions are given every year, writes,

> Oncologists today encourage second opinions, and everyone gains confidence on hearing that a decision has been endorsed by another. Cancer is a disease for which the "first shot" is the most important, and you want to feel confident when you begin a treatment that it is, indeed, the one that offers the best outcome.

STAYING NEAR HOME

When Sarah M. was diagnosed with non-Hodgkin's lymphoma at age 56, she was thankful she was married to Herb, a physician. He could understand all they were hearing about possible treatment options and could then explain them to her.

"There was this sense of urgency to do something," Herb said, "all mixed up with the emotional reactions we were experiencing because of the diagnosis. It helped to be able to look things up on the Internet. All sorts of Web sites were available."

"It was wonderful to have Herb," Sarah said. "There were times when I couldn't read even one more piece of information. It was just too hard. But he could read it and filter the information down to what I really needed to know, and then I'd read that."

On the day her biopsy showed lymphoma, Sarah's surgeon called a nearby oncologist and got her an appointment for three weeks later. In the meantime Sarah and Herb studied their options. Their oncologist received good recommendations from people they trusted.

"We could have chosen to go somewhere far away," Herb said, "but doing so consumes energy, and it takes time. We knew our oncologist was on speaking terms with doctors at Johns Hopkins Oncology Center, and she could call them with questions. We didn't feel we had to run across the country to get the expertise we needed."

When they saw the oncologist, they both liked her. She decided on a treatment plan that minimized side effects, an important consideration for Sarah because she was just then setting up a new nonprofit organization. They also got a second opinion with a specialist at a cancer center several hours away, who confirmed the treatment plan.

"I think it was important to have a physician who felt comfortable with our getting a second opinion," Herb said. "She wouldn't have felt threatened if we'd decided to go somewhere else for the whole treatment, and in fact she offered to set up Sarah's appointments if we had gone that route."

Getting her treatment near home meant that life could stay as normal as possible for Sarah. "Being home meant that we had emotional and spiritual support available to us," she said. "When Herb wasn't available, friends drove me to my clinic visits. When I've been hospitalized, our friends and pastors—and, most importantly, our three adult children—can visit me. Healing, for us, means more than just what medicine can offer."

PROVIDERS OF CANCER CARE

Who are the doctors who care for people with cancer? Most people with cancer go to doctors who have taken years of specialized training to be a cancer doctor. After their training, they have to pass a rigorous examination offered by a "specialty medical board" in order to become certified. The number of cancer doctors (oncologists) who had been certified by four different specialty medical boards numbered more than 10,000 in 1997.

- the American Board of Internal Medicine—6550 medical oncologists

- the American Board of Radiology—1468 radiation oncologists

- the American Board of Pediatrics—1348 pediatric hematology oncologists

- the American Board of Obstetrics and Gynecology—568 gynecologic oncologists

Being "board-certified" is not necessary before a doctor can treat people with cancer. Some doctors treat cancer as well as a wide range of other diseases. In Italy, for example, cancer is primarily treated by general internal-medicine doctors and general surgeons. In many cases, cancer takes up half their workload.

Board certification is a relatively recent development, so a doctor who has been practicing oncology for many years may not be board-certified. Also, sometimes certification is not available. For instance, there is no board certification for surgical oncology. So a surgeon who has gone through special training and now operates only on people with cancer—and who does so extremely well—won't have a piece of paper that says "certified."

SEEKING A SECOND OPINION

Even though I was a doctor, what I knew about Hodgkin's lymphoma on the day I was diagnosed could have

fit inside a teacup. A few terms flashed through my mind—
"Reed-Sternberg cells," "MOPP"—because they'd showed
up on the multiple-choice certification exams I'd taken in the
past. But that was about it. I needed information—and in
the next few days I certainly soaked up stacks of lymphoma
facts. But far more than information, I needed a doctor who
had both information and experience. I knew that being 15
weeks pregnant made me "a complicated case." Don and I
wanted our baby to live. We knew I needed an oncologist
who focused on lymphoma—and we really wanted one who
had treated pregnant women before.

I lived in a town that had oncologists—and good ones—
but none that specialized in lymphoma.

Certainly it would have been easier to stay home. Just
thinking about having cancer made me feel panicky enough—
and adding the thought of traveling to a strange place to treat
it threatened to smother me. My local oncologist, Marshall
Leary, was also a trusted friend and an excellent doctor. On
the day my lymph-node biopsy showed cancer, he made room
in his packed schedule to meet with Don and me. He agreed
that a lymphoma expert—somewhere—would be best for
me. He or she would be able to suggest an effective treatment
for me that would also be the least toxic to our unborn baby.

Somewhere in America was the lymphoma specialist that
was right for me. But who? And where?

Once I'd made the decision to travel, the choices multi-
plied. We got on the phone. No—actually, Don got on the
phone. I'm afraid I wasn't much help in researching. I was
still overwhelmed at the thought of having cancer and
couldn't distance myself enough from my emotions to be
able to look rationally at the options. And time was ticking
away. Don made dozens of phone calls, and so did Dr. Leary.
A friend from medical school told Don about Carl Freter, a
lymphoma specialist at the Lombardi Cancer Center in
Washington, D.C.

Lombardi Cancer Center is a "major cancer center" by anyone's definition. It's one of a network of comprehensive clinical cancer centers designated by the National Cancer Institute (NCI).

There are 60 NCI-designated cancer centers scattered throughout the country. But Bruce Hillner, who has studied and written papers on how cancer gets treated, estimates that fewer than one out of ten people with cancer are treated at NCI-designated centers. One reason may be that those centers are clumped in a few geographic areas of the U.S.— especially in the Northeast and southern California.

In *The Complete Cancer Survival Guide* the authors list the "top cancer centers in the United States," adding 39 other hospitals to the 48 NCI centers that were designated at the time they wrote the book. Those 39 hospitals have ranked high in *U.S. News & World Report* magazine's annual rating of "America's Best Hospitals" for cancer care. This list broadens the choice for someone who wants to be treated at a major cancer center close to home. One of these 88 major cancer centers is within driving distance for the vast majority of Americans.

DECIDING ON A PLAN

Choosing Lombardi Cancer Center had other benefits for me. It was affiliated with Georgetown University, where both Don and I had gone to medical school, and near which we both still had friends. And flying to Washington, D.C., fit well with another key aspect of my life. Getting my cancer treated was my highest priority, certainly, but I was still the mother of two small children. My parents lived outside Washington, D.C., so we could stay with them and they could watch our children while Don and I were at Lombardi.

But—unless I absolutely had to—I didn't want to stay at Lombardi for my entire treatment. Don needed to get back to work, and I didn't want to be separated from him. Nor did I want to give birth so far from home. My church and most of my friends were back home. Couldn't I just be evaluated at Lombardi by Dr. Freter, have him figure out what would be the best treatment, and then get the bulk of my actual treatments back home?

The answer turned out to be "yes."

It could just as easily have been "no." When Lou Ellen Russell was diagnosed with a fast-growing breast cancer, her doctor recommended that she get treated at a breast-cancer center that was a five-hour drive away. She needed intense treatments, and she needed to receive them there. "I spent the summer in a hotel room," Lou Ellen said. "I didn't even have a car there. The cancer center picked me up for treatments twice a day."

But she doesn't regret that time. "I didn't have my friends bringing me casseroles and coming to visit me," she said, "as I would have had if I'd stayed home. And I missed my husband terribly. But it was a special time to be with God and learn more about him by reading the Scriptures and praying." Now, ten years later, she is cancer-free.

Choosing to Travel

Ten days after I first felt the enlarged lymph nodes, I was flying to Washington, D.C. I carried with me on the plane some slides of the cancerous lymph nodes that had been made by my local pathologist. Dr. Freter showed these to the pathologist at Georgetown to make sure he interpreted them the same way. I also brought actual copies of the few X rays I'd gotten by that point, in addition to the reports about the "reading" of those X rays by the radiologist. Since I had not been "staged" yet—meaning we didn't know how extensive my cancer was at that point—I needed a couple of days of tests to determine what stage my cancer was at.

Don and I both liked Dr. Freter from the start. Somehow he was able to combine active involvement in research with genuine concern for patients. When he talked about treatment options, he mentioned our unborn child—certainly the subject looming in my mind also.

Dr. Freter decided on a plan that involved monthly cycles of seven drugs and every-few-month follow-up appointments for tests back at Lombardi. He wanted to see how I responded to the treatment. I was given the first cycle of chemotherapy before I flew home.

Since then, I've asked Dr. Freter how typical my experience was. "Your situation happens fairly frequently," he said. "There's no simple way to categorize everyone's experience. A second opinion at a cancer referral center ranges from giving general recommendations to the patient's oncologist, to giving a very specific treatment plan to their doctor (either a primary-care doctor or an oncologist), all the way to completely taking over their care. There are so many factors to consider—interpersonal relationships, travel distance, the expertise of the physicians involved, and how medically complex the situation is."

ALLOWING FOR FUTURE FERTILITY

In the week after the September 11, 2001, terrorist attacks, I remember reading about other people who escaped from the World Trade Center towers. One story told of a husband and wife who led a small company with a dozen or so employees. Their first thought was to get their employees out of the building.

But before she left the office, the woman made a detour. She took the time—what was it? thirty seconds? a minute?—to remove the hard drive from their main computer. She carried it safely out of the building.

Because of her foresight, the company was able to continue its work, hardly missing a beat. That hard drive contained their company's past, and was thus the key to its future.

When people are diagnosed with cancer, they are seldom thinking about their fertility. Simple survival is their main concern. Yet on some future day—a day when their treatment for cancer is behind them and they are beginning to look forward—they may deeply regret not thinking about fertility at the time of diagnosis.

For cancer treatment often causes infertility. This won't bother those whose families are complete, but it is a critical issue for people who may want children in the future. Both chemotherapy and radiation can cause infertility, although—depending on the age of the person getting treated—it may be only temporary. Obviously, surgery to reproductive organs may lead to infertility also.

So, as distressing as it may be, the time of diagnosis is the time to think about fertility. For a man, this is a simple process of storing his sperm in a sperm bank before therapy begins. Sperm can be frozen indefinitely.

For a woman, the process is much more complex and, alas, more expensive. It also takes time because hormones must usually be given to stimulate her ovaries, after which the eggs are collected. This may lead to an unacceptable delay in cancer treatment. Also, if a woman is married, she may be offered the option to store embryos rather than just eggs. An embryo is formed when an egg and a sperm unite, and it is the beginning of human life. The future of each embryo, therefore, must be considered just as carefully as any other human being's.

Ignoring a Tornado

I remember those weeks after my diagnosis as a whirling, emotional blur. Only clinging to God kept me from sinking under the fear, and only because of God did I experience islands of calm.

A surgeon I know once told me about a woman who had come to him more than a year earlier because of a suspicious mammogram—there was a spot that looked like it might be cancer, but she'd need a biopsy to know for sure.

"I can't have surgery right now," she told him, "because I need to go with my husband on a business trip." He urged her to reconsider, but she left his office and didn't return for three months. She finally agreed to a breast biopsy, and it showed cancer.

Now he told her she needed to have surgery to remove the cancer and needed to see an oncologist. She refused both. "I'll come back when I'm ready," she said.

She came back to see him two months later, but still wasn't ready for surgery. She did agree to some tests to see whether the cancer had spread. It had. There was cancer in her other breast as well as in her lungs.

As my surgeon friend was telling me the story, his face stiffened and he paused. Then he said, "Two weeks ago, she died."

I've thought of that woman a lot—and of other people with similar stories. I've had patients who have ignored my pleas to get a follow-up on some worrisome test. Before I had cancer, I couldn't fathom why someone would postpone getting a firm diagnosis or vital treatment. But now I have a glimmer of understanding. Is the person grappling with a paralyzing fear? Maybe life is in such a delicate balance that acknowledging cancer would topple it over. Are there perhaps no family members or friends who would be understanding?

STAYING FOCUSED

I know that when I was first diagnosed, I needed help. I was too flustered to make calls to look for a lymphoma specialist—the phone calls that Don made. I didn't have enough energy to fly myself and two toddlers to Washington, D.C., on my own. Many people helped me get to a major cancer center to get the help I needed—and quickly—and I'm grateful for them all.

Don made sure that I was moving forward in the medical system so I could get the help I needed, just as Yin Liang and his co-workers made sure that everyone had left the office on the fortieth floor of One World Trade Center and that everyone was moving down the stairs.

On September 11, 2001, just like many people, I could barely function. I listened to my patients, examined them, wrote prescriptions—but my heart was in New York City. In between patients I'd take a few minutes to watch the horror on the television in the lobby. Since that day, whenever I've seen those same patients, I've scanned my "9/11/01" clinic note to see if I missed anything important.

On September 12, I started to wake up early—at 4 A.M.—but was still dreaming. In my dream I was racing down a stairwell full of people and panic and confusion. Down and down and down I went, always downward. Finally I shook myself fully awake. *All those lives lost,* I thought in the darkness. The reality of death pressed down on me.

On an early morning years earlier, the thought of death had also burdened my mind. It was April 6, 1994—the one-year anniversary of my diagnosis with Hodgkin's lymphoma. Just a few decades before I'd been diagnosed, people with Hodgkin's had quickly died. The average life expectancy at that time was one year. I remember thinking, *Without chemotherapy, today I would be dead.*

So as dawn broke on September 12, I found myself asking, *If I'd been in One World Trade Center yesterday, would I have left without delay? Would I have gone back to my desk to retrieve something? Once out of the building, would I have kept moving so I'd have been far enough away when it collapsed?* Those who swiftly decided to leave—and then stuck with that decision—were more likely to be alive a few hours later.

And when people learn they have cancer, having that same kind of focus might be just the thing that saves their lives.

If you have cancer...

Consider asking yourself these questions:

- Have I found an oncologist with skill and experience in treating my kind of cancer, or a physician who can coordinate my medical care?

- Have I followed through on the recommendations made by my physician? Are there any areas where I have been slow to respond or completely resistant? If so, why?

- Are decisions about further diagnostic tests being made quickly, and is the treatment plan being decided on? Is there anything I am doing to slow down the process? Is there anything that I can do to speed it up?

CHAPTER EIGHT

GETTING SPECIALIZED HELP

Quick decisions ✱ *Referrals*
Benefits of major cancer centers ✱ *Thinking about our resources*

IN THE ISRAEL OF 2000 YEARS AGO, tax collectors were hated. Matthew was Jewish, but he collected taxes for the Roman conquerors. The Romans didn't care how much Matthew collected—they just wanted their cut. So Matthew became rich at the people's expense.

But then he met Jesus. Jesus walked by and said, "Follow me."

So Matthew did.

Turning his back on the piles of money in his tax collector's booth—and slamming the door on ever being able to collect taxes again—Matthew got up and followed Jesus.

Matthew's life changed—instantly. His income plummeted, and he began roaming the countryside in the company of a homeless man. He abandoned his former life to pursue a new hope—a hope that was embodied in Jesus Christ.

QUICK TURNAROUND

Matthew responded quickly to Jesus' invitation. I admire him—I'm no Matthew. Unless I'm forced to think quickly, I take my time with decisions. And if forced to decide more quickly, I tend to become angry and frustrated.

Sometimes, though, cancer forces quick decisions.

When Evie made plans to travel from Oregon to visit her daughter and her family in Boston, she got an appointment for a routine checkup with the doctor whom she knew from the time she'd lived in Boston. But the doctor's exam led to an ultrasound and then—two days later—to surgery for suspected, and then confirmed, ovarian cancer.

"My surgeon was an oncological gynecologist," Evie said, "to whom I was referred by my original doctor. I didn't realize at the time how important it was to have a specialist in cancer surgery. Now I know I might have had to have a second operation if I hadn't had that surgeon in the first place."

She began chemotherapy at Dana–Farber Cancer Institute, a major cancer center, ten days after her surgery, and she ended up staying in Boston for all six months of chemotherapy. Her life had turned upside down, and she was far from home. "Still, it was less disruptive for me than it would have been for another person," she said, "since I was able to stay with my daughter and her husband and children. Also, I had a tremendous personal support system in Boston. I know I wouldn't have come through chemotherapy as well as I did without that support system in place."

The Possibility of Referral

Dr. Marshall Leary is my oncologist here in Monroe, Louisiana. When he begins to take care of someone with a life-threatening cancer, he almost always offers the possibility of referral to a major cancer center.

"We give the standard therapy here—what is standard across the country," he says, "and that's fine for common cancers. But if you've got a rare cancer, then you've got to get to a major cancer center."

If someone asks to be referred, even if the cancer is a common one, he always does it. "If you want to go, you need to go," he points out. "Otherwise, you'll always wonder what would have happened if you had gone."

He doesn't push people to go if they resist. "When I suggest such a referral, I get three responses. One: 'Yes, I'll go.' Two: "No way, I'm not going.' And three: 'My family wants me to go, so I'll go.' I think when people say their family wants them to go they really want to go themselves, but they're afraid it will hurt my feelings. But it doesn't hurt my feelings. And besides, they almost always come back to me to get their treatments."

WILL I BE JUST A NUMBER?

In a story in *Prevention* magazine about writer Gregory White Smith and his 14-year battle with a brain tumor—a battle he considers successful because of his willingness to travel to top-notch cancer centers—Smith is quoted as saying, "I'm stunned by the people who will drive 8 hours to see a nephew or 4 hours to see a football game but won't drive 2 hours to a major hospital."

When I was first diagnosed, one aspect of going to a major cancer center made me uneasy. Would there be so many other people at the center that my needs would get lost in the swirl? Would I be treated like a "number"? Lombardi Cancer Center is in Washington, D.C., the city where I went to medical school. But I wasn't used to city living anymore. Where would I even park?

I was relieved to know that the center had thought of issues like parking (they had an attached garage with reduced-rate parking) and hundreds of others. Registering, for instance, was a simple process. Looking back, I'm not surprised to know that major cancer centers have thought of the details that help smooth the way for new patients from out-of-town. They want me to go there—even if it ends up being only for a visit or two.

❧ EIGHT BENEFITS OF GETTING CARE AT A MAJOR CANCER CENTER ❧

A person may be able to walk two blocks to get to a major cancer center or may have to drive hundreds of miles. Do the "positives" of getting care there outweigh the "negatives" of travel, expense, and being uprooted? To see if the scale tips toward cancer centers, here are eight distinct benefits they offer.

BENEFIT ONE: STATE-OF-THE-ART TREATMENT

Major cancer centers are magnets for doctors who want to stay current with the most up-to-date therapies. Is it possible to stay current and *not* practice at a major center? Absolutely, yes. Any doctor can read about new treatments in medical journals and can attend conferences where the latest therapies are taught and discussed. Plus, a particular cancer may not have had any treatment breakthroughs for many years. Perhaps new therapies have been proposed, but they're no improvement over the old ones. In that case, any oncologist practicing anywhere is likely to be up-to-date. But someone practicing at a major cancer center has more frequent opportunities to hear the latest information—through lectures at "noon conferences," for example.

Doctors figure out better ways to treat patients with a certain illness by giving a large number of people a new therapy and comparing their response to a large number of people getting the established therapy. In the world of cancer, many of these studies originate at major cancer centers, and most of the people in them get their treatment there. More and more, though, oncologists in smaller medical communities are involved in carrying out the promising new treatments and studying the responses (see benefit seven).

It takes time for state-of-the-art therapies to radiate out from the halls where they have been discovered. Even when a new treatment is studied and plainly proven to be better, it may be years before all oncologists across the country adopt it. "A significant lag exists in achieving widespread use of the best therapies," note National Cancer Institute researchers. Using those "best therapies" saves lives. The NCI article states that "at least a ten percent reduction in mortality could be achieved through the widespread use of available state-of-the-art therapies."

A cancer doctor at a major cancer center is likely to know the most promising treatment for a certain cancer. That doctor may even have discovered it.

BENEFIT TWO: ACCURATE STAGING

Each kind of cancer acts differently, but each starts out small and grows over time. Experts have studied the pattern of growth for each different kind of cancer and have separated that pattern into stages. The stage of a person's cancer is a vital piece of information. The stage determines what treatments are suitable.

In general, people who are treated for cancer at a major center are evaluated more thoroughly than people treated at community hospitals. They go through more tests in an attempt to accurately assess how extensive their cancers are. Once doctors know the stage of a cancer, they can decide how best to treat it. For example, if they think they are treating a stage II cancer but it is actually a stage III, then the treatment is not likely to work.

Often, people end up being placed at a higher stage after they've had a further workup at a major cancer center. They were at that higher stage before they went there, of course, but no one knew it. What a blow it is to hear that a cancer is more advanced than previously thought! But knowing the truth benefits the person with cancer. A stage III cancer needs a more aggressive treatment plan than a stage II cancer. Through the benefit of accurate staging, no time is wasted with a futile treatment before the person gets what is appropriate.

BENEFIT THREE: HIGH VOLUME

High volume? What does this mean—a blaring radio? No, by "high volume" I mean people—the number of people treated or operated on. The more people served at a medical site, the better the outcomes tend to be. "Where organizational factors have been assessed, the predominant relationship is between higher volumes and better outcomes, particularly for complex surgical procedures."

I'm not saying that, for instance, each of the 93 people treated for prostate cancer in a certain year at a major medical center will have a better outcome than each of the 11 people treated at a community hospital. It's just a general trend. The less common the cancer, or the more difficult the surgery needed to remove it, the better the outcome tends to be at a place with "bigger numbers."

Several studies have shown this same trend with high-risk cancer surgeries. These are surgeries that require a lot of technical skill, and there's a high risk of complications and setbacks in the recovery period. In the report *Ensuring Quality Cancer Care*, published in 1999 by the Institute of Medicine's National Cancer Policy Board, two studies of such high-risk surgeries are described. They both show fewer postsurgery deaths in high-volume hospitals compared with low-volume hospitals.

This report also describes studies that show better outcomes at high-volume hospitals for men with prostate cancer needing extensive surgery and for women needing breast-cancer surgery. Other studies show better outcomes when people need complicated chemotherapy strategies, such as bone-marrow transplants.

The overall goal of *Ensuring Quality Cancer Care* was to recommend to U.S. physicians ways to improve treatment of cancer. In its conclusion, the report makes ten specific recommendations to improve care, the first of which is,

> Ensure that patients undergoing procedures that are technically difficult to perform and have been associated with higher mortality in lower-volume settings receive care at facilities with extensive experience (i.e., high-volume facilities). Examples of such procedures include removal of all or part of the esophagus, surgery for pancreatic cancer, removal of pelvic organs, and complex chemotherapy regimens.

The more complicated people's medical needs are, the more they benefit by going to a high-volume hospital.

BENEFIT FOUR: DOCTORS TALKING WITH EACH OTHER

My daughter's fourth-grade class was peppered with high achievers. Each wanted to be the top student—to grasp new math concepts the most quickly, to get the most "points" in the book-reading program, to have the highest grades on tests. Martha Grace studied hard—there was peer pressure to keep up, and she did well. Likewise, a major cancer center is peppered with high-achieving cancer doctors. There is peer pressure to stay up-to-date with the latest treatment recommendations, and most do.

Having a cluster of cancer doctors all in one location means they talk with each other about the people they are taking care of. If a doctor's treatment plan develops a glitch, another doctor might have dealt with something similar, and a quick dialogue in the hallway might provide an answer. Most cancer centers have regular "tumor conferences" also, where specific treatment plans for specific people are presented. I remember attending these when I was a medical student, and I learned a lot from the lively (and sometimes heated) discussions. The human body is so complex that every possible response to a treatment can't be predicted—and when doctors stay connected with other doctors it keeps everyone sharp.

BENEFIT FIVE: A TEAM OF DOCTORS

A woman with breast cancer might need surgery, radiation therapy, and chemotherapy. But which to do first? It depends on exactly what the cancer looks like under the microscope, whether it has spread, and how quickly it seems to be growing. And in the course of her treatment the woman will need a surgeon, a radiation oncologist, and an oncologist—but who should coordinate her care?

At a major cancer center those three doctors are liable to see themselves as part of a team. The patient may have other long-term illnesses—such as high blood pressure or diabetes—complicating her care. Other doctors or health professionals will likely be part of the team, and together they'll weigh all the options. Ideally, one doctor will stand out as the woman's main contact, the one who integrates all the options into a single treatment plan.

BENEFIT SIX: A LEARNING ENVIRONMENT

Most major cancer centers are connected to medical schools and serve as places where young doctors receive their training after medical school (as residents). This means that medical students and residents will be roaming the halls and may be involved in the care of people with cancer. If they're not too overworked, they can be very helpful.

When I was a medical student, I was assigned to a small number of patients. This enabled me to find out details of their lives that helped me serve them better. I like to talk with people, and always have. In a discussion with other doctors on whether a man could be discharged home, I'd pipe up, "He lives in a second-floor apartment, and his only son is in Cleveland." Or, to explain a low potassium level, "She doesn't take her potassium every day because the pill is too big."

The benefit went both ways. I learned more about diseases by following my patients than books could have ever taught me. And I learned about people, too, and how they respond emotionally to being sick.

I remember one man I followed for several weeks when I was a third-year medical student. He had a malignant melanoma that needed to be removed from his back—his third melanoma skin cancer in a decade. It was removed, and then the spot was skin-grafted. He was often hurting, but he welcomed my presence when I came to check on him. I helped explain things his doctor had said that he didn't understand, and if he asked a question that stumped me, I hunted down the answer. He helped me develop as a doctor, and I helped him get the medical care he needed.

BENEFIT SEVEN: CLINICAL TRIALS

Years ago, cancer research was done in only a few large medical centers. To be part of the research, people with cancer either had to live nearby or be willing to travel to the medical center—and then stay there. Many saw this as a last resort. But this is no longer the case.

Now doctors across the entire United States are conducting cancer research. It takes time and energy—more time and energy than simply treating people with cancer takes—so not every oncologist is involved. But until everyone is perfectly satisfied with all available therapies—and no one is—doctors will be plunging forward with new ideas. Clinical trials are the way those new ideas are tested.

Seventy out of every hundred children who develop cancer become part of a clinical trial. Granted, cancer is relatively rare in children. But the participation of so many people in clinical trials has led to an explosion of successful treatments for childhood cancers. During the time span from 1960 to 1990, the percentage of children who were alive (and essentially considered cured) five years after being diagnosed with a solid tumor jumped from 28 percent to 70 percent. Dr. John Lukens from Vanderbilt University School of Medicine, writing in 1994, attributed that advance to clinical trials. "The process is labor intensive, tedious, and expensive, but over time, it has paid big dividends. Without question, clinical trials are the driving force behind the successes of the past 3 decades."

Among younger adults (ages 20 to 49) with cancer, only four out of a hundred participate in clinical trials, and among older adults (50 and up), less than two out of a hundred participate. The National Cancer Institute helps to pay for the bulk of clinical trials—1200 as of December 2000, involving 23,000 people with cancer. Most of these trials are based in a major cancer center, but there are also hundreds of affiliated community doctors who enroll people and follow them through their treatment.

People who join clinical trials aren't helping just some anonymous person who will get cancer sometime in the misty future. They are very likely to benefit themselves. A study of children in a clinical trial found that children in both arms of the trial—both the new-treatment arm and the standard-treatment arm—had improved survival compared to children who were not part of the clinical trial. This may be partly because people in clinical trials are followed closely and any problems are taken care of quickly.

Also, by the time most people get involved in a clinical trial, the trial is in "phase III." Phases I and II have made sure the new treatment is reasonably safe, and now it is being compared with the established treatment. "Phase III trials study drugs that have proved to be effective treatments in Phase II trials and that appear to be as good as or better than standard treatments for a particular tumor." The new treatment may be buried treasure—and the people in a phase III trial are among the first ones to discover it and profit from it.

BENEFIT EIGHT: OTHER PROFESSIONALS

Nurses in a major cancer center are more likely to have received extra training in cancer—maybe even in particular types of cancer, such as female cancers. Or they may be very comfortable taking care of people who are having bone-marrow transplants. Being specialized makes these nurses better able to deal with problems as they come up.

Doctors and nurses aren't the only ones who care for people in a hospital. Social workers connect people with agencies that can meet their needs, and they help smooth the way to discharge. Chaplains visit people and ask if they would like to discuss issues of spiritual or emotional concern. Nutritionists assess what people are eating, compare that with what they should be eating, and then make recommendations. Counselors and psychiatrists work with people who are struggling emotionally.

Major cancer centers are not the only places where social workers, chaplains, nutritionists, and mental-health professionals are available to help. Almost all hospitals have these—and other—supportive professionals. But a major cancer center will have a greater number of them, and they're likely to have a better understanding of the particular problems that people with cancer go through.

BARRIERS TO QUALITY CARE

All cancer care is not equal. Cancer is expensive to treat. For people with scant extra income—and for the uninsured—top-notch cancer care may be beyond reach. Even for people with health insurance, some costs of care aren't covered. Researchers in Texas have studied how lack of money creates a barrier to getting cancer treatment. "This research shows the need for staff at cancer treatment facilities to be aware that there are nonclinical, financial factors that are important considerations in the treatment of cancer patients." Transportation is essential. "Patients, particularly minorities, may opt to forgo needed care in the absence of available and affordable means of transportation to treatment facilities."

Various agencies—nationwide and local, faith-based and secular—are poised to help people with some of the costs of getting cancer care. Getting connected to that help means taking time to make inquiries—an effort that may be extremely difficult for a financially strapped person.

Also, people older than 65 are more likely than younger folks to receive less aggressive—and less effective—cancer treatment. Several research studies have shown this trend. This is probably a combination of doctors' underestimation of how much treatment older people can tolerate and older people's unwillingness to receive certain treatments.

BENEFITS AND COSTS: CONSIDERING OUR RESOURCES

In medicine, almost no decision is purely right or purely wrong. Making a decision is a balancing act. Are the possible benefits worth the possible costs? For some, the possible benefits of a referral to a major cancer center will be obvious and convincing. For others, they will be unclear.

Deciding to get evaluated—and possibly treated—at a major cancer center takes personal resources: energy, money, effort. Some people diagnosed with cancer don't have these resources. Others have them, but may choose not to use them to go to a major cancer center. But newly diagnosed people should understand what the benefits and costs of going to a major medical center could be. They should feel free to bring the subject up with their local oncologist. And if their oncologist brings the subject up before they do, they need to carefully consider what is said.

And after considering the options, they may come to realize that their resources are more plentiful than they'd thought they were.

If you have cancer...

Consider asking yourself these questions:

- Has my doctor offered to refer me to a major cancer center? If so, and if I did not accept that offer, why not?

- If my doctor has not offered referral to a major cancer center, have I brought up the issue? If not, why not?

CHAPTER NINE

MAKING DECISIONS
IN PARTNERSHIP

Partnership with doctors ❧ *Making a personal connection*
"The three C's" ❧ *Empathy*

FIFTEEN YEARS AGO, when I'd been a doctor for less than a year, Don and I visited the Old Court House Museum in Vicksburg, Mississippi. In 1863, during the Civil War, Vicksburg was under siege for 47 days before it finally fell to General Ulysses Grant. The museum was packed with fragments of Civil War history. I expected that. But I didn't expect to laugh.

Encased behind the glass of one display was a bullet—an ordinary-looking bullet. The story of the bullet, typed neatly on a card, came from a medical journal article that a Dr. L.G. Capers had written in 1874. In May of 1863 he'd been a surgeon in a brigade that had fought at the battle of Raymond, slightly east of Vicksburg. During the battle, that bullet—so he wrote—had hit both a soldier and a young lady. It seems it had passed through the reproductive organs of the former and entered those of the latter. The 17-year-old maiden then became pregnant from that bullet.

By this point Don and I were laughing, but it got even better. Nine months later Dr. Capers "delivered this same young lady of a fine boy." The doctor then introduced the young parents to each other, and they were married before "the little boy had attained his fourth month." They had a happy marriage and had more children—conceived in the ordinary way.

What fun! Medically that was so unlikely that it was virtually impossible. And to have it "happen" to two eligible youths added to my doubts. "But do you think he was being serious—maybe to save the reputation of their families—or was it a big joke right from the beginning?" I asked Don.

"I don't know," he said. "Why don't you ask the lady at the gift shop?"

So I did. I was smiling when I asked my question, but she stared at me so sternly that I stopped smiling. "What are you trying to say?" she asked.

I swallowed. "Did people back then think that could really happen?" I asked in a small voice.

She sighed. Like a schoolteacher speaking to a dull student, she explained, "My dear, that was a *doctor* who wrote that account."

"But..." I said—then I stopped myself. Her face was unyielding. I finished the sentence to myself. *So what if he was a doctor? I'm a doctor, too, and that story is bunkum.* Instead, I forced myself to nod. "I see," I said.

"Well, then," she concluded crisply, and she turned back to her work.

A doctor had written the story. That made it true. *A doctor is the ultimate authority.*

Partnership or Paternalism?

I've thought about that woman countless times over the past 15 years—usually when I'm taking care of someone who reminds me of her. I'll be explaining various options to a woman patient, for instance—laying before her a choice between an expensive once-a-day antibiotic or a cheaper one that must be taken three times a day. And she'll say, "Oh, Dr.

Givler, you choose. You know what's best. Just tell me what to take." Then the lady from the museum shop in Vicksburg will flash into my mind. *A doctor is the ultimate authority.*

In such a case, since the person sitting before me needs me to be an authority, I'll be one. I'll choose which antibiotic to prescribe, or determine that her arthritis has progressed to the point that she needs a hip replacement, or decide that she should take a pill every day to prevent migraine headaches. But I'm uncomfortable with that. In decisions such as these—not life-and-death, but significant—I much prefer that my patients tell me their preferences and let me know what side effects and inconveniences they are willing to tolerate. I prefer partnership over paternalism.

Sometimes, though, being an authority has its advantages.

I remember seeing a man for his second visit a few years ago. "And how much are you smoking now?" I asked.

"I stopped."

"How great!" I said, looking back at my notes from the first visit. "Last month you told me you smoked two packs a day."

His eyes grew large, and he looked perplexed. "But you told me to quit," he stammered, "and so I did."

"That's right," I said quickly. "I told you to quit, and so you did. Of course you stopped smoking. Right, right." I sat quietly on my stool, but inside I was jumping up and down. *He quit! He quit! When I told him to quit, he did!*

I wish all my smoking patients would see me as an authority when it comes to their smoking habits. Well, they don't, but—just in case—I tell them all to quit.

THE PATTERN OF DISILLUSIONMENT

I rarely have the "problem" of patients who trust me too much, though. Few doctors do. Most people come to see me for the first time with an attitude of guarded suspicion, not of unqualified trust. Many people carry wounds from previous encounters with doctors. But this is not really new. In A.D. 399 the theologian Augustine wrote, "The man who has tried a bad doctor is afraid to trust even a good one."

With authority comes great responsibility. Some doctors have abused their authority—perhaps by seeking their own financial gain at the expense of their patients' health—and the people they injure stop trusting them. No problem there. Those particular doctors have shown themselves to be untrustworthy. The trouble is, sometimes those injured people stop trusting any doctor. Then, when a crisis comes (such as being diagnosed with cancer), they have a wall of mistrust to break down before they can establish a "therapeutic relationship" with the doctor who takes care of them.

What is a "therapeutic relationship"? It happens when there's an atmosphere of respect between doctors and patients—an atmosphere that is positive enough to allow a free flow of communication. The patients tell their doctors what is important to them, and they ask questions. The doctors listen. The doctors tell the patients about their illness and what they can do to help themselves. The patients listen. Such an atmosphere fosters good health care.

I've taken care of people who, the first time I saw them, kept their arms crossed and shook their heads in time with everything I said. In such cases, I know I need to give these people time to trust. So I spend much more time listening than talking, and I try to communicate that I care. After several visits, we've usually developed enough of a therapeutic relationship to allow me to do more talking.

If, once they trust me, I ask those patients about their previous experiences with doctors, they'll typically tell a story of holding a particular doctor in high estimation. Then the doctor did something selfish or uncaring that crushed them. Now, in their view, all doctors are tarnished. I grab that opportunity to point out that all doctors—including me—are capable of being selfish and uncaring. We are humans. Humans fail other humans. We've been doing so for thousands of years.

When the stakes are low, taking whatever time is needed to develop a therapeutic relationship makes good medical sense. But when the stakes are high—such as when a person has cancer—doctors feel an urgency to plow forward with treatment suggestions, whether or not the person is in emotional harmony with them.

People with cancer benefit by having a therapeutic relationship with their doctors. It's worth the time it takes to develop one. Four centuries before Jesus Christ was born, the Greek physician Hippocrates observed, "Some patients, though conscious that their condition is perilous, recover their health simply through their contentment with the goodness of the physician."

The Doctor as Partner

Judy G. learned she had breast cancer after a routine mammogram in 1994. As soon as she was diagnosed, she asked many friends—some who were medical professionals, some who had been treated for cancer—whom they would recommend for a cancer doctor. She knew she wanted one with whom she could develop a therapeutic relationship. Though only 43, she had already been battling two other chronic diseases for several years. She'd had her share of doctors she didn't trust.

Friends recommended an oncologist who sounded like someone she could work with. "It helped that he also had a stellar reputation in my area," Judy said. "That meant I came to my first appointment with a measure of trust—and that trust was confirmed during his first candid discussion with me."

Judy wanted to be an active partner in dealing with her breast cancer, which she realizes not every woman wants. "I've heard that some doctors hesitate to be totally honest and open because they aren't sure how much the patient really wants to know. So I knew I needed to initiate the partnership—letting him know that I see myself as part of the treatment team."

Her doctor told Judy all her options, laid out possible outcomes and side effects, and informed her how everything might affect her two other chronic diseases. She ended up having a lumpectomy followed by seven weeks of radiation therapy. "I felt like I developed a partnership with my oncologist. He was the expert regarding the cancer, but I was the expert on my own body and my emotions. A team approach was crucial for me."

THE CORNERSTONE OF GOOD DOCTORING

In her book *The Human Side of Cancer*, Dr. Jimmie Holland talks about "the three C's." They are *competence, compassion,* and *caring*—and she calls them the cornerstone of good doctoring. "Competence" is the ability to accurately diagnose and effectively treat illnesses. "Compassion and caring" involve the awareness of another person's distress and the desire to reduce it.

"A competent doctor without compassion or caring is daunting to the patient feeling uncertain and vulnerable," she observes. But didn't doctors enter medical school with not only a love for science, but also a desire to help people? Yes, Dr. Holland writes. "Most young people go into medicine with a strong sense of humanity and humility, with the three C's strongly in place. But something happens to many in medical school as they cram in more and more facts: They become fatigued and think they lack time for considering the human side of illness."

Most doctors eventually return to their original vision of caring for people—although that vision may be buried under the stresses of office management, family life, finances, and the need to stay up-to-date in medical knowledge. How to unearth that vision? There are ways, and patients can help.

MAKING A CONNECTION

Just as some doctors are comfortable making medical decisions without much input from their patients, some patients are very comfortable not giving that input. But this doesn't mean they don't want any information. They may not want a detailed explanation of every side effect of a treatment, but they probably want—in broad brushstrokes—a sense of what to expect.

Likewise, some doctors feel far more comfortable when their patients take an active role in their own treatment decisions, and some patients want to know everything possible—though probably not all at once. Our brains need time to absorb new information—and everyone's brain is unique in how much it can handle, and how quickly.

A *British Medical Journal* article put it this way:

> Research has indicated that the vast majority of cancer patients want to be informed about their illness. However, it is also recognized that patients vary in how much information they want and that this may change during their illness. These attitudes are reflected in the efforts that patients make to obtain further information or to resist information that is offered to them.

When Sara M. was diagnosed with myelogenous leukemia, she had arrived home from her honeymoon only ten days earlier. Her doctors quickly agreed that the best treatment for her would be a bone-marrow transplant—involving at least a month of intensive treatment in the hospital. Sara agreed, but she didn't want to hear about every possible complication. She is a basically upbeat person and wanted to stay that way. "I could hardly process anything in the beginning," she says. "There was a lot of information I didn't want to hear. I didn't even want it in my brain."

But she couldn't go through a bone-marrow transplant without being informed of the risks and signing a consent form that said she had. "When she came with the consent form, I told her I only wanted to hear what she absolutely had to tell me in order to sign it," Sara said. "So she paced it slowly, asking several times whether I could handle what I'd already heard. In the end, I could sign the paper."

When there's a match between what a doctor feels comfortable telling and what a patient feels comfortable hearing, the patient is far more likely to be satisfied with the encounter. If there's a mismatch, all is not lost.

If, say, a woman wants more participation in decision-making than her doctor initially welcomes, she can say, "I want to hear all my options, and what you are thinking as you make decisions. Also, I may sometimes bring information I get from other places for you to look at, and it's really important to me that you consider it." Both doctor and patient may be stretched, but openness in communication will keep both of them from becoming frustrated.

In an article by Harvard Medical School researchers, the authors quote a cancer doctor as saying,

> What you do get from talking to people—the questions they ask and the way they conduct themselves—is how much the person wants to know. We want patients to have a good understanding, especially if we are going to be treating them. We need them to be kind of partners in what we are doing. So although we don't bludgeon people with the truth, I...would like each

patient to have the fullest understanding of the disease they can tolerate.

BECOMING WELL-INFORMED

When journalist John Hill was diagnosed with prostate cancer in August 2000, initially he panicked. At 55, he had already outlived almost all the men in his family—men who had all died of cancer. But then, though still anxious, he set out to learn everything he could about his cancer and how to treat it. In a remarkable series of articles in Monroe, Louisiana's newspaper, the *News-Star*, John detailed every twist and turn in his path to knowledge. Finally he settled on a treatment plan. "Once the tension of deciding what surgery and what surgeon was over, I immediately felt a calm and peace that I haven't felt, almost since it began. The tension of waiting for reports on your cancer and choosing among the various treatment options is very stressful."

He was informed—but not in charge. His relief came from knowing he was in good hands.

Even oncologists who are diagnosed with cancer shouldn't manage their own treatment. Sir William Osler, who taught medical students in the wards of hospitals a century ago, declared that "a doctor who treats himself has a fool for a patient." This maxim was hammered into my head during my years of medical training. Everyone needs someone who can take a step back—emotionally—and look at the whole picture.

An important 1991 article on doctor–patient communication, called the Toronto consensus statement, states the following:

> Explaining and understanding patient concerns, even when they cannot be resolved, results in a significant fall in anxiety. Greater participation by the patient in the encounter improves

satisfaction and compliance and outcome of treatment....The level of psychological distress in patients with serious illness is less when they perceive themselves to have received adequate information.

I know that when I understand the reasoning behind a piece of medical advice, I am much more likely to comply with it.

THE SECRET OF MEDICAL CARE

Seventy-five years ago doctors were taught to govern all decisions on behalf of their patients. I'm glad those days are gone. But 75 years ago most doctors knew their patients well. Maybe they'd taken care of their patients' parents, too, and also took care of their children. Most decisions made by doctors were in the context of understanding the rich backdrop of their patients' lives and relationships.

But even back then, people admitted to a teaching hospital were likely to have a doctor who didn't already know them as a person. In 1927 Dr. Francis Peabody wrote an article, "The Care of the Patient," that has been required reading in many medical schools. He urged student doctors to realize that a patient's emotional life will affect his physical life—whether or not his disease is serious. Students must seek to establish "that intimate personal contact between physician and patient which forms the basis of private practice." And then he concludes,

> The good physician knows his patients through and through, and his knowledge is bought dearly. Time, sympathy and understanding must be lavishly dispensed, but the reward is to be found in that personal bond which forms the greatest satisfaction of the practice of medicine. One of the essential qualities of the clinician is

interest in humanity, for the secret of the care of
the patient is in caring for the patient.

Today's doctors and patients have more obstacles to
establishing a therapeutic relationship than Dr. Peabody ever
dreamed of. Immeasurably more medical facts are sloshing
around doctors' heads, and time pressures are intense. Getting to know a patient's family is hit-or-miss in a large hospital setting.

The "house call" is no longer a routine part of health care,
but I look back at the era of the house call a little wistfully.
Doctors learned so much about people by seeing them in their
homes. They could see their patients' living situations, their
positions in their families, and their support systems. I'm sure
it made it easier to recommend treatments— they knew what
advice they could realistically expect a person to follow.

BECOMING THREE-DIMENSIONAL

But what about people with cancer? They have never met
their doctors before being diagnosed, and now there's no
time for each to get to know the other in a leisurely way
before treatment must begin. True. But there are ways to
speed up the process.

Sara M., whom I mentioned earlier as having myelogenous leukemia, knew she wanted to establish a relationship
with her doctors and nurses before she took the plunge of a
bone-marrow transplant. She wanted to be known, and there
wasn't much time. So she threw a party.

"I reserved one of the conference rooms in the hospital
and invited all the doctors and nurses. I served little sand-
wiches and gave out little Christmas ornaments as gifts—it
was right before Christmas," she said, then laughed. "People
still talk about it, three years later. 'Oh, you're the girl who
had the lunch.'"

She became known, all right, and that made it easier for her to bear the weeks in the hospital for the transplant. But in the party she got to know her doctors and nurses as people, too. It went both ways.

As a doctor, when people show me photographs of people who are important to them, I get a sense of what their life is like outside the clinic. A photo takes only a few seconds to look at, but it can communicate volumes. Getting a note from a patient—saying thanks, or sharing some news—helps me better grasp who he or she is as a person, also.

And what about gifts? I hesitate to mention gifts because I never really understood why my patients gave me gifts until I got sick myself. I valued the givers' thoughtfulness, but I didn't understand their motivation. Were they trying to sway me in some direction? But that changed when I got cancer. Now I understood. I was so intensely grateful for my doctors' help in keeping me alive that I gave them all gifts. And ever since I've been a better gift-receiver.

I'm not showered with gifts, but I've received books from a fellow book-lover, fish from a fisherman, eggs from a farmer, and a painted teapot-shaped sign from a craftswoman. These speak to me of our bond as patient and doctor, yes, but also of the individuality of the giver. I look beyond the gift to the person who gave it—and this is possible because the gift reflects the giver's personality.

WANTED: Empathy

Some doctors have more empathy than others. Empathy has been defined as "the feeling that 'I might be you' or 'I am you,' but it is more than just an intellectual identification; empathy must be accompanied by feeling." Doctors need empathy to connect with their patients—whether they have a lot of it or just a little.

Of course, a completely empathetic doctor wouldn't be able to make rational decisions. If the patient were to begin to sob, then the doctor would begin to sob also. No, that wouldn't be helpful. Doctors have to distance themselves emotionally to some degree—otherwise they wouldn't be able to keep seeing patients. They'd be exhausted, for one thing. They don't have to allow everyone they see to seize their heart—but they can allow each person to touch them.

Marcia G. was diagnosed with breast cancer when she was 11 weeks pregnant with her third child. She then had surgery, several cycles of chemotherapy before her daughter was born—healthy—and then chemotherapy and radiation afterwards. "Regarding the obstetrician and the oncologist," Marcia says, "I found them to be very nurturing. Everyone was really concerned about the baby. My oncologist seemed to just love his job. He'd play a little game with me when I got chemo. I'd say, 'This will keep the cancer from coming back, right?' and he'd smile and say, 'That sounds reasonable. I think you're right.'

"The radiation oncologist wouldn't play that game, though," she continued. "He always wanted to give me statistics, but I didn't want to hear them. I just wanted him to agree with me that the cancer wouldn't come back."

As Marcia demonstrated, humor helps develop the bond between doctor and patient. Anger, though, hinders it. When someone directs fierce anger my way, I have a hard time penetrating that anger so I can see the person behind it. I'm not saying that angry people must pretend that everything is beautiful. If something is displeasing, it needs to be expressed. But there's a big difference between saying heatedly, "How could you do this to me, you awful person!" and keeping a steady voice and saying, "What you just did makes me very angry. I would like to know your reasoning behind it." With words like those, the incident can be discussed and dealt with.

DIFFERENT FOLKS

Not every encounter with a doctor will be a building block for developing a therapeutic relationship. Sometimes a doctor is frantically busy, or needs to focus urgently on the patient's physical problem, or is distracted by a personal family problem. If this unsatisfactory encounter is not customary, then it can be viewed as a small glitch in the path to connecting with a doctor.

Sometimes, though, it becomes clear that a doctor is not ever going to express much empathy—and that the relationship between doctor and patient will never get down to the level of feelings. What to do then? Maybe—accept it. The depth of a partnership I'm willing to accept with a surgeon who is well-known for his technical skill, for instance, is less than what I'd like with an oncologist I'll be working with for many months. There are some surgeons who are warm and thoughtful, certainly, but many more have little interest in making a personal connection with their patients.

Many of the same skills used in developing a relationship with a friend also apply to making a connection with a doctor. Kind words should go both ways, and as Mother Teresa said, "Kind words can be short and easy to speak, but their echoes are truly endless."

If you have cancer...
Consider asking yourself these questions:

- Do I want my doctor to make most of the decisions for my medical care, or would I rather be a partner with him or her in making those decisions?

- Have I been hurt by a doctor in the past? If so, am I carrying over a feeling of mistrust into my current interactions with doctors?

- Can I think of a way to make a connection with my doctors so they can better see who I am as a person?

CHAPTER TEN

FACING FAMILY AND FRIENDS

Seeking support ❋ *Taking a risk*
How families are affected ❋ *Teamwork*

MOSES LED THE CHILDREN OF ISRAEL out of Egypt. A tough job for anyone, let alone an 80-year-old man—especially since his task wasn't over. Now he had to make it through the wilderness—a wilderness full of danger.

He didn't do it alone. He had family, and he had friends.

Good thing, because right away he faced opposition. Men from the tribe of Amalek attacked. Moses sent Joshua to lead the fight against them, while he himself held up the staff of God on a nearby hilltop. "As long as Moses held up his hands, the Israelites were winning, but whenever he lowered his hands, the Amalekites were winning."

What a responsibility! I can't keep my arms raised even 20 minutes—especially not holding a staff—and winning a battle takes a lot longer than that. But Moses had help. Aaron, his brother, and Hur, his friend, had come up the hill with him. When his hands started drifting downward, the two other men seated Moses on a rock and helped his hands stay up—one taking the right one, and one the left. By sunset, Joshua had defeated the Amalekites.

Moses wasn't alone. When his strength wasn't enough, Aaron and Hur stepped into the gap.

People with cancer aren't alone, either. Somewhere in their lives they have an Aaron-like family member and a

Hur-like friend who can step in when their own strength wilts.

Before an Aaron and a Hur can help, though, they have to know there's a need. And that can be hard to express.

It was certainly hard for John Hill. Communication shouldn't have been hard for him—he's a newspaper journalist, after all—but, though his prostate biopsy had been scheduled for nearly three weeks, he didn't tell his wife about it until the night before. "I didn't want to worry her," he later wrote in one of his series of *News-Star* articles. "I tell myself it's because she [has a stressful job]. But the real reason was I didn't want to think about it."

He later found out the consequences of keeping his feelings bottled up—they burst out in harsh ways against blameless people. So in the weeks that followed he wrote about how he learned to express his fears and to accept help. Things went better after that.

SUPPORT AND SURVIVAL

There's good reason to seek out support. The stronger the social and family relationships, the better the chance of responding to cancer treatment and surviving. One large study done in California showed that people with fewer social connections had poorer survival rates. Another study done in Wisconsin revealed that married people had improved survival over unmarried people—even after adjusting for the fact that unmarried people tend to be diagnosed with cancer at a more advanced stage.

Although that study showed better survival in married people overall, it was more true for men than women. For a woman, it seems, whether the marriage is stormy or peaceful makes a big difference. That is, the quality of the relationship is key. A medical textbook, *Cancer and the Family*, reports, "It can be shown that distressed relationships may outweigh the positive effect of social support." Another study of women with breast cancer found that the women who had a large number of supportive friends, relatives, and neighbors (more than 11 total), or who had three or more special friends they could call on for help, were more likely to be alive four years after diagnosis.

What kind of support do people with cancer want? There are five different types of support:

1. *information*—helping a person with cancer find out the facts relating to their illness

2. *practical help*—giving tangible assistance: a meal, baby-sitting, a car ride to the doctor's office, money

3. *emotional support*—being available when a person wants to share inner thoughts and feelings

4. *affirmation*—communicating that a person is still valued and respected—cancer hasn't changed that

5. *network support*—a group of people with common concerns that gives support to everyone in it

People with cancer are helped by all five kinds of support—though not all at once. They cannot expect every kind of support from each person they know. Could one person even provide all five kinds? I doubt it.

Sara M. didn't think so either. After she was diagnosed with leukemia at age 29, she grew closer to both of her sisters. But what she needed from one was very different from what she needed from the other.

"One sister was more emotional, and the other less so," Sara said. "Some days I'd want to talk to someone who would worry, so I'd call the emotional one and tell her about how hard life was. Other days I'd need to hear my other sister say, 'Tell me only about the good things going on in your life.' I'd call one or the other depending on what I needed at that point."

Letting People Know How to Help

Sometimes people don't know what to do or what to say. They're afraid their attempts to help will wound instead. Their loved one—the person with cancer—needs to let them know how they can help.

Marcia G. did just that. When she was diagnosed with breast cancer—while pregnant—she knew her husband would be supportive in a practical way, and he was. He did much of the child care for their two- and five-year-olds, and made life as easy as possible for her. But she also knew he was the kind of person who didn't dwell on unpleasant thoughts and wouldn't try to guess what she was feeling.

"Early on I realized I needed to give him some direction," Marcia said. "So I told him very specifically what I needed: extra hugs and touching, and a sympathetic ear when I needed to talk about something—even if he wasn't worried about it himself."

Marcia was asking for emotional support. Pinpointing her request made it easier for her husband to give her the support she needed. Another time she asked him for another form of support—affirmation. "I asked him once, 'When you look at me, do you see a fat bald-headed freak with one breast, or do you see the person you married?' He didn't hesitate. 'The person I married,' he said. That was great. And I was especially glad he didn't hesitate."

Feeling Vulnerable

Asking for help is risky. People might help—or they might not. I can't force people to help me. Sometimes they won't, and sometimes they can't.

Elizabeth Sherrill was a young mother when, in 1957, her husband was diagnosed with malignant melanoma, a fast-growing skin cancer. She and John were both writers for *Guideposts,* a Judeo–Christian magazine, but at that time they were not people of faith themselves. After John's surgery, Elizabeth reached out to her grandfather, with whom she'd always been close.

"Both our fathers were gone by then, and I didn't yet know my heavenly Father," she recently wrote in *All the Way to Heaven*, a book about her journey to God. "The day after the surgery I poured out to him my fears, the uncertain prognosis."

But her grandfather responded with a recital of his own illnesses, his own needs. "It was a growing-up passage for me," Elizabeth recalls, "just when so much growing up was asked. To see Papa not as I needed him to be, but as the central figure in his own story....In time it meant a deeper, more adult love for him, but that night it was another of life's props knocked away."

She later describes how this terrible time "without props" was an important step in her finding a greater good—faith in Jesus.

One of my patients, Joy D., already knew that "greater good" at the time she was diagnosed with non-Hodgkin's lymphoma. In fact, she thinks she leaned on God for help just as much as she leaned on family members during the difficult early months of treatment. When she felt herself getting discouraged, she went first to God.

"I knew my loved ones were deeply affected by the cancer, too," she told me, "and if they saw me in depression about it, it wouldn't help them. If I stayed 'up' about it, it helped them. So I asked the Lord to help me, and he did."

OTHER FAMILY MEMBERS STILL HAVE NEEDS

Family roles often shift when someone gets cancer. That shift may be barely noticeable, or it may be massive. A wife and mother, for instance, may be the pivotal member of the family. Her husband and children depend on her for emotional support. If she gets cancer, everyone in the family is deeply affected. As she goes through cancer treatment she can no longer meet everyone else's emotional needs, now that her own physical and emotional needs are mushrooming. The way that family functions will have to change—at least temporarily—if everyone's needs are going to get met.

How can families make the shift? Here are some key ways:

* *Talking about it.* Open communication means that each family member knows how everyone else is being impacted.

* *Seeing this time as a challenge.* A family that faces a challenge together is likely to grow stronger as a unit.

* *A new normal.* Life may never "get back to normal." Instead, there will be a new "normal." Acknowledging that is the first step to adjusting to it.

* *Dealing with conflict.* People often think that ignoring problems will make them go away. Instead, problems that aren't dealt with tend to get bigger and drive people apart.

* *Accepting outside help.* If a family functioned well before cancer intruded, it can be hard to admit that it's no longer true. The easiest kinds of help to accept from non–family members are information and practical help.

THE YOUNGEST ONES AFFECTED

Open communication is doubly hard when a parent with cancer has children he or she is still raising. Parents want to be available for their children's needs, yet going through cancer treatment drains them of the energy they'd like to be pouring into their children's lives.

I remember not wanting to tell my children I was sick when I first learned I had cancer. They were very young—still toddlers—and I wanted to shield them from any anxiety. I didn't want them to think I couldn't take care of them. And what could they understand, anyway?

But Don reminded me that children understand more than we parents realize, and that we needed to be able to discuss my cancer openly in the future. They knew something was different—their routine was being disrupted. Telling them later would only be harder. So we sat them down and told them in simple words that I was sick and needed lots of treatments to get better. They took it in stride.

Older children need to be told too, though now that my children are older I can see how hard it would be to tell them. Even as I tried to deal with their struggles, I'd be dealing with my own—

* I want to be the one to raise them. Will I be around to see them grow up?

* Kids ask tough questions that we adults tend to suppress. Will I be able to answer them without bursting into tears?

* Will they bring up issues that I don't feel ready to deal with?

Children look to their parents to model how to deal with painful situations. *If Mom talks about the cancer, it must be safe for me to talk about it, too. If I ask Dad a simple question and he answers it, maybe I can ask a deeper one—the one that's really bothering me—next time.*

Talking to kids about difficult situations is important, even if they're not obviously upset. They want to know that their needs will still be met. Or they may be angry or scared and not know how to express those feelings. Very likely they have gaps in what they understand—and using their vivid imagination, they've probably filled in those gaps with misinformation.

Children don't have the big-picture perspective on life that adults do. If something traumatic happens in the family, they tend to see themselves as responsible. They're quick to take the blame if things don't work out as well as everyone has hoped.

True, parents shouldn't promise their children that "everything will be back to normal soon." Though they'd like it to be, they can't make it happen. But parents can say,

This is not your fault.

We are upset, but we are not mad at you.

We care about your needs, and we want to meet them.

We want to answer your questions as well as we can—whenever you're ready to ask them.

We love you. Cancer hasn't changed that.

THE STRAIN ON THE SPOUSE

When I was diagnosed with cancer, my world came crashing down. But not only mine—Don's world would never be the same, either. I'd leaned on him for emotional support ever since we were married, but now he almost had to *carry* me. And—though I was oblivious to the fact at first—he had his own struggles.

He didn't want to lose me. I'm sure that, partly, he dreaded being a father of motherless children, but he knew he'd also miss my companionship and the history we had shared. Furthermore, his job at the hospital hadn't changed—he still needed to do the same amount of work there—yet his job at home had expanded.

"I was frightened," Don has since told me. "For most people who are facing cancer and are frightened, it's the fear of the unknown. But for me, it was a fear of the known—because I had some sense of what lay ahead for our family, and it wasn't pretty."

Our eleventh anniversary came two days after I was diagnosed. "I remember thinking, *This could be our last anniversary,*" Don said. "We'd always talked about sitting in rocking chairs on our fiftieth anniversary while listening to the waltz they played at our wedding. But now that scenario was uncertain. Life wasn't going according to plan."

I had cancer, but in practical ways my life had gotten easier. I obtained a leave of absence from work. Friends brought meals. I took naps. If I said I didn't have the energy to change a diaper, Don did it. I must admit I was tempted to never again "have the energy" to change a diaper—but I knew I shouldn't test the limits of Don's love. And besides, I loved him and knew he was doing so much for me. To the extent that I could, I wanted to lighten his burden.

All our friends and family were concerned about me. I know Don was the one that kept them informed about what was happening to me. That was a full-time job in itself. Mary Jo Fisher is a doctor whose husband was diagnosed with colon cancer at age 59. In a recent *Journal of the American Medical Association* she writes,

> It is almost inconceivable how much time and work it is to have a loved one in the hospital. I thought I knew this, but I really didn't fully appreciate it before. As a physician, I was the appointed spokesperson for all of our relatives....Each family member needs a detailed account, education to enable understanding of the situation, and continual updates and reassurance.

Through the months of her husband John's cancer treatment 45 years ago, Elizabeth Sherrill also suffered, right along with him. Because of that, she has since developed "a lifelong empathy with the partner in a crisis—the competent, smiling, supportive one with the hollow place inside." When one partner in a marriage gets cancer, two lives are uprooted.

UNDERSTANDING DETACHMENT

Years ago, many people thought cancer was contagious. Few people believe that myth today, but a stigma still remains. Some see people with cancer as unclean somehow, or as having failed—failed to stay healthy, I guess.

At the time I found out I had cancer, I had a lot of friends. I have a lot of friends still. Many of my "pre-cancer" friends are even better friends today. But some are not. Some of them pulled away when they found out I had cancer.

I've thought about that a lot and have tried to figure out why. I don't like to lose friends. But I think I understand now—and I mostly accept it.

Some people simply don't know what to say to someone who shares "bad news." Others feel so grieved at the sight of suffering that they avoid it. Being around someone whose life is threatened is too scary. Still others feel that they are no longer able to relate to someone who has cancer—they now live in two separate worlds.

Alice Trillin wrote about this experience in a 1981 article adapted from a talk she gave to doctors. Four years earlier she had been diagnosed with lung cancer.

> I didn't feel different, didn't feel that my life had radically changed at the moment the word *cancer* became attached to it. The same rules still held. What had changed, however, was other people's perceptions of me. Unconsciously, even

with a certain amount of kindness, everyone—
with the single rather extraordinary exception of
my husband—regarded me as someone who had
been altered irrevocably.

Cancer is also a blaring reminder that "human existence
is but a breath." Sometimes people try to avoid reminders
that life is brief. A person with cancer might be that reminder.

Lola N. understood that reality when she was diagnosed
with ovarian cancer at age 62. "After my first surgery the
surgeon told my family I had only three months to live. I
remember how people were afraid to come see me in the hospital—I think they were afraid of my reaction to being 'terminal.' And one nurse was amazed that I was still cheerful.
I heard that she asked someone else, 'Doesn't she know she's
terminal?' But I didn't know how someone who is terminal
is supposed to act. We're all terminal. We just don't know
exactly what time." Lola is right. Five years later, she's still
alive.

Cutting Grief in Half

I will always remember the friends who reached out to me
and my family when I was going through cancer treatment.
I didn't want to meet new people—unless they'd had cancer
and had an inkling of what I was going through—but I definitely wanted to see my already-established friends.

And so many did reach out. Friends brought meals, ran
errands, and offered to baby-sit our children. Friends I'd
made in college visited from Boston and Dallas, as well as my
cousin Chris from California and my sister from New York.
I found myself agreeing with Francis Bacon, who said that
friendship "redoubleth joy, and cutteth griefs in halves."

I remember how hard it was to admit that I was needy
enough to require all this help. But helping me helped the
people who felt so bad that something so wretched had happened to me. They could do something to make my life

easier. As Oscar Wilde said, "If a friend of mine...gave a feast, and did not invite me to it, I should not mind a bit.... But if...a friend of mine had a sorrow and refused to allow me to share it, I should feel it most bitterly." By allowing others to help, I was helping them.

I could actually have hurt my family and friends if I'd kept my troubles to myself. This was made clear to me a couple of years ago when I saw a patient of mine, Beatrice W., who uncharacteristically was anxious and very sad. It turns out her sister had recently died of breast cancer. They had been close. I probed further, and I learned that her sister hadn't told her about the cancer until a few days before her death. Beatrice knew she hadn't been feeling well because her niece, who was still at home, had said that her mother had been spending a lot of time in bed. But Beatrice's sister had sworn her daughter to secrecy—a terrible burden for a teenage girl.

Her sister's death threw Beatrice's entire extended family into chaos. *How could they have not known? What could they have done to help her?* Two years have now passed, and Beatrice is still grieving deeply. I know her sister would have chosen differently if she could have seen how much pain her decision would cause.

TEAMWORK TRIUMPH

When I heard Beatrice's story, it reminded me of another story. A man carrying a 60-pound backpack is offered a ride home by a friend. "You can put your backpack in the trunk," says the friend as they approach his car.

"Oh, no," says the man, keeping his backpack on his back. "Your bringing me home is nice enough. I wouldn't want you to carry my backpack too."

A man going through cancer treatment may need to be "carried" for a while. If so, he needs to toss that backpack in the trunk.

For remember that Moses could do what God was asking him to do—hold up his arms over the battle in the valley below—only with the help of his brother and his friend. He needed them. As the writer of the book of Ecclesiastes says, "Two are better than one, because they have a good return for their work: If one falls down, his friend can help him up. But pity the man who falls and has no one to help him up!"

Standing together with their family and their friends, people can triumph through the experience of cancer.

If you have cancer...
Consider asking yourself these questions:

- Do I find it hard to ask for help? What category of support do I need (information, practical help, emotional support, affirmation, or network support)? When people offer to help, can I point them toward one of these categories?

- How is my family handling my having cancer?

- Are some friends drawing closer, and are others pulling away?

CHAPTER ELEVEN

COPING WITH TREATMENT

Rest, food, and exercise ❧ *Trusting*
Dealing with side effects ❧ *Finding support groups*

ELIJAH WAS A POWERFUL PROPHET of God in Israel, but on that particular day he was exhausted. Totally spent. Drained. When I read in the Bible how he spent that day, I'm sure of it. First Kings 19 tells the story: Elijah had just sensationally defeated the prophets of the god Baal—whom most of Israel worshiped—and had then prayed for the end of a three-year drought. After that, he ran down from the mountain where he'd been and all the way home—ahead of the rain that was beginning to pour out of the sky.

I would think the king of Israel would have been impressed with such evidence of God's power—but I would be wrong. The king remained furious at Elijah, and he stirred up his wife Jezebel's anger against him, too. And she promptly let Elijah know that she was about to send hit men to kill him.

What did this dog-tired prophet of God do? He started running again—this time for his life. Two days later he collapsed under a juniper tree and asked God to let him die. "I have had enough, Lord," he said. "Take my life." But God didn't continue the conversation. Yes, he wanted to talk with Elijah, but he knew Elijah wasn't ready yet. Instead, he allowed the prophet to lie down and sleep. After a while,

God sent an angel to wake him up and give him fresh-baked bread and water. Elijah ate, slept again, and then ate another angel-provided meal. When he woke up the second time, he was refreshed, and he wanted to live. He was ready to hear what God wanted to say.

When he had reached that juniper tree, Elijah had been physically and emotionally depleted. Is it any surprise he cried out in despair? But God knew what he needed, and it wasn't instruction or information. "Instead," Marilyn Yocum writes, "the angel made sure Elijah received two things: adequate rest and proper food."

Targeting Dividing Cells

Cancer treatment is rough. For me, chemotherapy felt like an attack on my body—and in a sense it was. The medicines were designed to wipe out rapidly dividing cells. Ideally, only cancer cells would have been affected, but unfortunately any dividing cell was fair game. After all, the cancer had begun with one of my normal cells going haywire and dividing without restraint. How could the medicines distinguish between cancer cells and my normally functioning cells, if both were dividing? So with every treatment, some of each were destroyed.

This took a toll on my body. Not only did it have to perform its normal functions, but it also needed to replace all the chemotherapy-damaged cells. When broken apart, both the good and bad cells alike released their fragments into my bloodstream. My body then had to dispose of them, which took work.

In my case, I was also growing a baby. My body was expending energy to allow him to develop inside me. And a lot of my emotional energy was centered on him, too. Would he survive this exposure to harsh drugs? Before chemotherapy, I'd been reluctant to take even a Tylenol for a headache, lest it harm him. Would God protect him from the chemotherapy?

OBSTACLE #1: FATIGUE

How did my body respond to all this? With fatigue.

It was as if my body were saying to my brain, "Hey, brain, I'm overworked down here. I can barely keep this ship afloat as it is. You'd better not ask me to do anything else that requires energy." But I, the mother of two active toddlers—someone used to pushing myself even when tired—kept trying to keep up my normal schedule.

The result was predictable: My body refused to cooperate.

It started out slowly—a day or two of sluggishness after each chemotherapy treatment, like walking through waist-high water. By the third month, though, I was a total blob for four days. Just getting up from a chair to get something in another room was a major effort. Thankfully I wasn't hurting anywhere, but I had a deep, penetrating tiredness. All I really wanted to do was to go to bed.

By my sixth month of treatment, I was no longer pregnant. God had kept my baby safe through chemotherapy and birth, and he was healthy and at home. This meant, though, that I was now the mother of a newborn—a newborn who didn't think that nighttime was a particularly good time to sleep.

I wanted to force myself to keep up, but whenever I did I started feeling nauseated and my body ached. Viral and bacterial infections plagued me. I learned to pace myself to do only the most essential tasks. Friends and family pitched in and helped in countless ways. People who loved our family took over most of my household responsibilities. Even now when I think of their sacrifices, I thank God for them. Don got up with our baby most nights. He was doing his job and mine, too.

Yet even as I knew I needed help, my inability to care for my family gnawed at me. Did my family no longer need me? Would I ever be useful again?

And the fatigue deepened. During those last three months, for several days after each treatment I had what I would call "flat days." I'd make myself get up and get dressed, but then I would collapse back in bed. For much of the day, I would lie as still as a stone, thinking for many minutes about tiny movements—how I needed to turn over, for instance—before I'd make myself do them. I was aware of each breath in and each breath out—for even breathing seemed to be draining me of energy.

SOLUTION #1: REST, HEALTHY EATING, AND—YES— EXERCISE

When my body was at its weakest, I needed to give it what it demanded: *rest.* Only rarely did I need to spend the day in bed, though. Other days I just rested for brief periods. I took naps most days.

Too much rest worked against me, though. If I slept too much during the day, I wasn't able to sleep at night. If I stayed active during the day, my nighttime sleep was more restful. These are well-understood "good sleep habits."

Some of my fatigue was due to anemia—that is, having fewer red blood cells flowing through my bloodstream. Red blood cells carry oxygen, which all tissues need, to every part of the body. Anemia is a very common side effect of cancer treatment. Two different times I was given shots of erythropoietin, which increased my red-blood-cell counts. Both times my energy level rose also.

Healthy eating was also important. I remember my body craving fruits, vegetables, and bread made out of whole grains. Chicken, fish, eggs, and milk products gave me the protein I needed. When I ate these foods, I felt better. Our bodies need nutrients to function well, but so many of the foods that Americans eat—and which are available everywhere—have few nutrients. We call nutrient-poor food "junk food." When someone's body is getting treated for cancer, it needs nutrients more than ever before. Now is the time to give the body what it needs.

I did not *exercise,* but now I consider that a mistake. Recent research has shown that when people being treated for cancer get regular physical exercise, they are better able to keep up with the ordinary activities of life. Their outlook on life improves also.

One study done in Germany showed that all it takes is 30 minutes of muscle movement a day. The researchers divided 60 hospitalized people with cancer into two groups. One they encouraged to exercise every day and one they didn't. The exercise was rhythmic and repetitive—similar to pedaling a bicycle. All then received bone-marrow transplants. At discharge, the people who exercised had less fatigue and fewer physical complaints than the non-exercisers. They also had less anxiety and mental distress.

It may seem odd that the way to get more energy is to use energy. That's why doctors have traditionally urged fatigued people to rest. But our muscles need to be moved if they are going to stay in condition. And because so much of the body's energy is going toward getting rid of the cancer, making muscles move takes more effort than it did before cancer treatment. So what many people do—as I did—is not move their muscles. But then their muscles become even *harder* to move. The result? Fatigue. "It is clear that lack—and even fear—of physical activity contributes to a self-perpetuating condition: diminished activity leads to easy fatigability, and vice versa."

On my flattest of flat days, I couldn't have exercised. But on most of the other days I could have taken a brisk walk. I wish now that I had been in better physical condition when I was undergoing treatment. Just a daily walk would have helped. Bike-riding or swimming would have, too. Looking back, and considering what research has shown, I know that exercise would have prevented some of my fatigue.

Today, I'm in better shape than I was then. Now I make myself exercise. Moving my muscles helps to increase my stamina and clears my brain so I can better focus on what I need to do. But I'm no athlete. I still don't find exercising irresistible.

OBSTACLE #2: ANXIETY

How did my head respond to chemotherapy? With anxiety.

I felt so vulnerable. I was taking medication that lowered my number of white blood cells, the infection fighters in my blood. When they were particularly scarce, I needed to take extra precautions to avoid germs. The few bacteria on that doorknob might not affect someone else, but they could make me sick. Or that friend's head cold might be insignificant for her, but if I caught it I might end up in the hospital taking intravenous antibiotics. So I washed my hands frequently and was always vigilant—always alert to the possibility of infection.

Midway through my months of chemotherapy I went to a seminar sponsored by a local hospital on how to cope with cancer treatment. One speaker in an otherwise excellent series of talks was an oncologist—not mine—who painted a bleak picture of chemotherapy, saying, "It's just a poison we're putting in the body." He reminded me of Winnie the Pooh's grouchy friend, Eeyore.

The lady seated next to me—who was going to start chemotherapy the next week—began to cry. Tears filled my eyes also. But I reached for her hand and whispered, "It's not that bad. Ignore him," and I stopped listening. I didn't need to accept another person's gloomy outlook if it sapped my morale and increased my anxiety.

For there were enough anxiety-producing events in my life going on without my looking for more. Before my baby was born I worried whether he would survive chemotherapy. I'd feel him kick and be relieved, but just 15 minutes later I'd be wondering if he'd died in the meantime. Then he was born—and after that I worried that he'd die in his sleep. I remember getting up to check on him a number of times some nights.

And I wondered if our house would burn down. Or if our children would get hit by a car as they crossed the street. Or if I would die—crossing the street, or in a plane crash, or because of a reaction to a chemotherapy drug—and they'd have to grow up without me.

I think these thoughts came because there was no margin in my life to allow for further disaster. I was already so close to the edge of my ability to cope. If another sudden sadness happened, would I crumble? My mind painted every possibility in catastrophic brushstrokes.

Also, I wasn't in control of my life. Now I was realizing I'd never truly been in control—but I sure thought I had been. Now so many aspects of my life were completely out of my control.

SOLUTION #2: CHOOSING TO TRUST GOD

When anxious thoughts rushed at me, I had a choice. I could dwell on them—or I could deal with them. And since I was anxious about things that were out of my control, dwelling on them wouldn't resolve them. I couldn't guarantee they wouldn't happen then, just as I can't guarantee they won't happen now.

The more I wallowed in anxiety, the more I got sucked downward. I needed help. I turned my thoughts to God. He knew what was happening to me, and I knew he loved me. And so I talked to him—telling him how I was feeling and what I was anxious about. *Everything looks dark here, God. Help!*

Something that author Elisabeth Elliot wrote in her book *A Path Through Suffering* helped me repeatedly. "Open hands should characterize the soul's attitude toward God— open to receive what He wants to give, open to give back what He wants to take." I'd think about that when my hands were clenched.

I'd peel back my fingers and lift my open hands to God. *Okay, Lord, I'm looking to you. I know there's a bigger picture for my life than what I can see right now. And I know you are here with me.* I needed to look beyond my current weakness and focus on God.

There were some things I *could* control, and doing them helped me shove anxious thoughts out of my brain. I listened to my body, and when it demanded rest I gave it rest. I tried to get good nights of sleep. I ate healthy foods, thus keeping myself focused on doing what I could to benefit my body. And exercise? Exercising would have helped, too, I'm sure. Exercise seems to help everything.

When I kept my mind busy with practical matters, both fatigue and anxiety shrank. Spending time with my husband and children calmed my mind—taking walks, reading books out loud, singing. Since my energy was limited, I let nonessential household tasks slide. Writing in my journal restored my energy like nothing else, and it also helped me sort out my thoughts and make sense of what was happening to me. Putting my fears down on paper made them seem more contained—and more manageable.

Medicines are available for both fatigue and anxiety, but they have their own set of side effects. I already felt like my bloodstream was a toxic soup, and so I wanted to add as few ingredients to it as possible. But if my doctor had strongly recommended that I take such a medication, I would have carefully considered it.

Disrupted Plans

Cancer treatment seldom goes according to the original plan. It certainly didn't for me. My head knew this before I started treatment, but my heart wasn't ready for it when it happened.

After six months of chemotherapy treatments, I thought I was through. But my checkup showed that the tumor—though tiny—was still shrinking. My oncologist thought it was probably just scar tissue, but maybe—just maybe—a cancer cell or two was still alive. He told me I needed two more months of treatment.

I was crushed. Thanksgiving and Christmas were approaching, and I'd been making plans for them. Now all I could plan for was being a blob. Each treatment drained me of energy. My thinking—once sharp and focused—was fuzzy and getting fuzzier. I didn't trust myself to drive, and I had trouble focusing on simple arithmetic.

Was my brain gone? Would my energy ever return? I had to trust that the first question's answer was "no" and the second's was "yes."

I told myself that these extra months of cancer therapy were an investment—like putting money in the bank. It was a brutal investment, true, but it would "pay off" in the future with restored health.

Side-Effect Gumbo

Everyone's cancer journey—at least in regard to side effects—is different. A hundred people could get the exact same surgery, chemotherapy, or radiation, and respond in a hundred different ways. I refused to read a list of all possible side effects to every drug I was given—I would have panicked. Instead, I glanced at the list and figured I'd read carefully about a side effect only if I actually experienced it.

Still, there are some common side effects that I knew I should be alert to, and I knew I should be aware of how they are usually treated. And the good news is that most side effects can be very effectively treated.

- *Nausea.* Ten years ago, people getting chemotherapy listed nausea as the most universal—and the most unpleasant—side effect. No longer. Medicines to block nausea—Zofran and Kytril—are given routinely, and they are remarkably effective.

- *Poor appetite.* When a person doesn't feel like eating, both the treatment and the cancer itself can be the culprit. But the body needs food to stay strong and withstand the battering of cancer treatment. It's hard to make yourself eat when you're not hungry, but it could mean the difference between thriving and barely surviving. Many cancer survivors first learn about good nutrition when going through treatment—and then they benefit from that knowledge for the rest of their lives.

- *Pain.* Not everyone with cancer experiences pain. People who do can be treated. All cancer pain can be made manageable, if not completely eliminated. Taking pain medication to treat pain is not a sign of moral weakness, and it's extremely unlikely to lead to addiction.

- *Depression.* Depression is not fatigue and it's not anxiety. It's not just feeling sad because life has taken a difficult turn. It's a deeper sadness and lethargy.

Depressed people seldom feel pleasure, and their sleep isn't normal. A major depression is a medical condition that interferes with healing, and it needs to be treated just like any other serious medical problem.

* *Less interest in sex.* I admit I didn't think much about sex when I was going through chemotherapy. But I was still married, and though Don was long-suffering, he still had needs. When one member of a couple has cancer, either spouse can bring up the subject.

* *Hair today...*From the beginning I decided I'd lose my hair gracefully. *Becoming healthy again is worth losing my hair,* I told myself. I bought a wig and several hats before starting chemotherapy. "Losing my hair will not bother me," I told Don. "My hair can be gone *forever* if it means I can live."

  Hah! So I *said.* When I started to lose it, though, I mourned its departure. Being hairless made my cancer so obvious—I couldn't blend into the crowd.

  I didn't actually lose every single strand of hair, although my hair became sparse. Having some wisps allowed me to wear hats instead of my wig (which itched). I combed the wisps forward so they peeked out of my hat.

One nice thing: Scant hair meant I didn't have to buy shampoo. One small bottle lasted all year.

SUPPORT—IN PERSON AND ONLINE

My family and friends gave me lots of support, but I still longed for a connection with other people who had cancer. The more their cancer was like mine, and at the same stage of treatment, the better. I wanted to be part of a support group. I didn't have the opportunity to join one until just before I finished chemotherapy, though. But even then it became pivotally important to me.

Our support group met weekly and had some members who'd been on the cancer journey longer than I had, and some shorter. We had a leader named Brenda, a caring and insightful social worker. Having a leader was important. She made sure the atmosphere stayed encouraging, and she kept us on track.

Internet support groups didn't exist in 1993, but I think I'd have joined one if they had. I know that a lot of people these days are getting some of the support they need while sitting at their computers—and people with similar cancers that are at similar stages can find each other. But for me, I don't think it would have matched the value I found in being with other flesh-and-blood people in the same room.

THE YEAR THAT VANISHED

The year I spent going through cancer treatment—and recovering from it—was not delightful. But it was endurable. There were even snatches of high-energy moments—times when I felt decent. I grabbed them. I used them to think through tough issues, to write in my journal, or to connect with my friends through letters or phone calls.

But when the energy wasn't there, I concentrated on the essentials. I didn't need to spend my precious energy struggling against the inevitable. This time would pass. The time of restoration would come.

As Lewis Sperry Chafer (the founder of Dallas Theological Seminary) said, "We still live in bodies with limitations, and all of us are subject to the circumstances of life. Neither should we mistake worn nerves, physical weakness or depression for unspirituality. Often we need sleep more than prayer, and physical recreation more than heart searching."

If I'm going through as life-threatening a time as the prophet Elijah faced, I need to lie down under the same juniper tree he did. And once I'm lying there—exhausted— what I need is sleep and nourishing food. After I'm refreshed, I'll be ready to reflect on the deeper issues.

If you have cancer...
Consider asking yourself these questions:

- How much exercise am I getting?
  What can I do to get more?

- Are the foods I eat good for me?

- Am I being swallowed up by anxiety?
  Can I look to God for help?

- Are there sources of support I can
  start developing now?

Chapter Twelve

Sensing a
Spiritual Dimension

Belief in God ✹ *Living out a belief*
Health benefits of religion ✹ *Experiencing God's love*

MY FAVORITE CHARACTER in Herman Melville's novel *Moby Dick*—and he is a *character*—is Queequeg. Once a Pacific-island cannibal, and now a harpooner on the same whaling ship as the book's narrator, Ishmael, Queequeg has always intrigued me. He is strong and uncivilized, yet noble and deeply spiritual. He is an unwavering friend to Ishmael, saving his life more than once.

So when Queequeg himself was so sick with a fever that death seemed inevitable, I was grieving along with Ishmael. Queequeg even had the ship's carpenter make him a coffin. But then he surprised everyone.

> But now that he had apparently made every preparation for death; now that his coffin was proved a good fit, Queequeg suddenly rallied; soon there seemed no need of the carpenter's box; and thereupon, when some expressed their delighted surprise, he, in substance, said, that the cause of his sudden convalescence was this;—at a critical moment, he had just recalled a little duty ashore, which he was leaving undone; and

therefore had changed his mind about dying: he could not die yet, he averred.

I think Melville intended this to be funny. A desperately ill Queequeg simply decided he had something to live for, and so he lived! I always chuckle when I read that. But I think Melville was reaching for a deeper truth also. He was contrasting the mystical power of Queequeg's convictions with Ishmael's rootedness in the material world.

Queequeg and Ishmael were opposites in so many ways. They shared friendship, but not faith. Ishmael, though technically a Protestant Christian, considered his religion just a superficial shell. Queequeg's faith impacted his life. No, even more than that—Queequeg's faith *was* his life.

Remembering that he had left a task undone was enough to boot Queequeg off his deathbed. He was a man of his word—his integrity was as much a part of him as the tattoos that covered his body. Mere illness couldn't keep him from his commitments.

Is "Wanting to Live" Enough?

Can that happen today? Can someone—no matter how sick—just decide to get better and pop out of bed? Should we doctors encourage our patients to all remember some undone task?

We may not need to. Most doctors can recall a time when a patient outlived all expectations so he or she could attend a wedding, a graduation, or a bar mitzvah.

But—and this is a big "but"—it's not just a matter of wanting to live. I'm thinking of two friends I met in a support group at a time when all of us in it were going through cancer treatment. These friends fiercely desired to live—far more than I did, I remember thinking at the time. But they didn't live. I felt each of their deaths like a blow. I was ashamed over still being alive. Didn't they deserve to live because of how much they wanted to?

And each of them believed in God and had asked him for healing. Why didn't God heal them?

I don't think God gave me back my life as a reward because I believe in him and love him. He loves me, I know, and he loved my two friends from the support group. I think he intends to do me good, whether I end up healthy or not, alive or not. I can't force him to keep me alive. God's just too big for me to use him as a "lucky charm."

"An Unfailing Stream of Energy"

When I was attending medical school, no one encouraged me to find out what my patients believed about God. That struck me as odd. My faith in God affected my own life in so many key ways—it seemed like we doctors were missing a crucial aspect of our patients' lives.

All that is changing. More than half of U.S. medical schools now offer courses that teach future doctors how to address the spiritual dimension of their patients' lives. Medical journals frequently carry articles on spirituality these days.

But practicing doctors have long known that believing in God impacts people's health. Way back in 1910 Sir William Osler wrote about "the faith that heals," stating that "nothing in life is more wonderful than faith....The one great moving force which we can neither weigh in the balance nor test in the crucible—mysterious, indefinable, known only by its effects—faith pours out an unfailing stream of energy while abating neither jot nor tittle of its potence."

According to Gallup polls, more than 95 percent of Americans believed in God in 1995—the same percentage as in 1944. And almost all of them consider their religion to be "very important" or "fairly important" in their lives. In fact,

72 percent say they "agree" or "strongly agree" with the statement, "Religion is the most important influence in my life."

But religion's "being important in my life" might not mean that my day-to-day decisions stem from my beliefs. I have some friends who believe in God and who try to find out what God wants for their lives. Then they try to do it. I have other friends who never think this way. They don't look for God to help them choose the direction their lives will go in.

INTRINSIC OR EXTRINSIC?

The two different ways my friends live show the difference between *intrinsic* and *extrinsic* religion. Back in the 1950s, psychologist Gordon Allport defined these two approaches. People whose religion is intrinsic, he wrote, "find their master motive in religion....Having embraced a creed, the individual endeavors to internalize it and follow it fully. It is in this sense that he lives his religion."

People whose religion is extrinsic "are disposed to use religion for their own ends,...to provide security and solace, sociability and distraction, status and self-justification. The embraced creed is lightly held or else selectively shaped to fit more primary needs. In theological terms the extrinsic type turns to God, but without turning away from self."

Writer Jean Fleming touched on that difference when she reflected on Jesus Christ's teaching about God in Matthew 6:33: "Seek first his kingdom and his righteousness, and all these things will be given to you as well."

> What does it mean to "seek first"? Certainly it does not mean sequence. It does not mean seek God first, then scratch that off the list and pursue the rest of life....Seeking God first is not a matter of *order*, but of *focus*.

> Christ must not become simply another item in our life—not even the most important item. He did not come in order to be the most crucial piece of our fragmented life; He came to absorb all of life—our family, job, talents, dreams, ministry—into Himself and impress on it His mark.

Ever since Allport first described the difference between "intrinsic" and "extrinsic" spirituality, other researchers have used these terms in their studies. One study done in 1991 looked at 103 women with breast cancer and found that the women with intrinsic religion were more satisfied with how faith helped them cope, when compared to those with extrinsic religion. Another done in 1998 surveyed 460 people at a family-practice clinic and found that participants with a high level of intrinsic spirituality had better overall health than those with a low level.

His Back to the Wall

When John Sherrill first learned he had cancer in 1957, he was a writer for *Guideposts*, a magazine that tells stories of how faith impacts people's lives. But faith had not impacted his own life—not yet.

He believed in God, certainly, and was "facing toward Jesus," but he had never made an internal commitment. His cancer was the worst kind of skin cancer—malignant melanoma—and fear hounded him. He was the father of three small children. But when the initial surgery appeared to have removed it all, John's fear melted away. All through those tense months, his level of involvement with God didn't change.

Then, two years later, the cancer came back. And it had spread.

"I thought I was going to die," John said, "and my doctor did, too. He told me to get my things in order because I had three months to live."

On the morning of the day he was to check into the hospital, John and his wife, Elizabeth, visited their neighbor, a Christian named Catherine Marshall LeSourd. Knowing he was about to have risky surgery, she asked him whether he believed Jesus was God. It was the key question, he knew, and one he'd never answered. He explained his reasons. But Catherine exposed the core issue.

> "You're trying to approach Christianity through your mind, John," she said. "It simply can't be done that way....You have to be willing to experience it first, to do something you don't understand—and then oddly enough, understanding often follows. And it's just that which I'm hoping for you today...that without understanding, without even knowing why, you say 'Yes' to Christ."

But he had reservations. His biggest one he stated frankly:

> It just didn't seem right to shy away all these years and then come running when I had cancer and was scared and had my back to the wall.
>
> "I'd feel like a hypocrite," I said.
>
> "John," said Catherine almost in a whisper, "that's pride. You want to come to God in your way. When you will. As you will. Strong and healthy. Maybe God wants you now without a shred to recommend you."

John left Catherine's house without answering the question she'd asked him, but struggled with it while driving home. Finally—as he passed a certain telephone pole he can still point out—he turned to his wife. "What do they call it:

'a leap of faith'? All right, I'm going to make the leap: I believe that Christ was God."

That decision had immediate consequences. First, he was relaxed as he faced surgery later that day, though the thought had earlier filled him with terror. And, most remarkably, the large lump of suspected cancer that had been there the day before had now shriveled to the size of a raisin—and it was cancer-free. John Sherrill believes that God healed him.

The decision he made on the day of his second cancer surgery shifted his spirituality from "extrinsic" to "intrinsic." If Christ was God, then he needed to live his life for him. In the years since, he has continued to be internally committed to Jesus.

✍ FIVE HEALTH BENEFITS OF RELIGION ✍

Not every person whose belief in God is "intrinsic" is healed of cancer, certainly. But the benefits are real, and doctors have begun to study them.

Three doctors who have for years studied religion's impact on health have written a comprehensive book, *Handbook of Religion and Health,* that pulls together and organizes thousands of research studies. The benefits that follow are gleaned from that book.

BENEFIT ONE: GREATER SOCIAL SUPPORT

The world's major religions all emphasize mutual support. Houses of worship are places where members give each other tangible and emotional support. Members don't have to rely solely on family members—if they have them—to help them when they need it.

Being part of a community of fellow-believers gives people a sense of identity. They are thus reassured of their worth. They are also given the opportunity to help others.

Reaching out to and encouraging others in worse circumstances is a powerful antidote to depression and other negative emotions caused by stressful life events. Altruistic behaviors help to meet others' needs, distract one from one's own problems, and promote feelings of usefulness, purpose, and well-being.

BENEFIT TWO: LESS DEPRESSION

Depression is a deep sadness that lasts a long time. Depressed people struggle to carry out the ordinary duties of life that others find easy.

People whose religion is intrinsic (that is, their belief in God helps to guide their behavior) are less likely than the average person to become depressed. "Even when these persons experience depression, available research suggests that they recover more quickly from it than those who are not religious." People whose religion is extrinsic (that is, they are motivated to be religious because of the benefits that religion brings) have *higher* rates of depression than the average person.

When life becomes stressful, the likelihood of depression increases. In the midst of a health crisis, those with an intrinsic spirituality are, again, less likely to become depressed. "Religious involvement plays an important role in helping people cope with the effects of stressful life circumstances."

When my patient Joy D., a woman with an intrinsic spirituality, was diagnosed with lymphoma, she instantly wondered if she was going to die. "But I had to leave that possibility in the Lord's hands," she said. "If I had dwelt on whether the cancer would take me, I would have become more and more upset, and would have probably fallen into depression. Then that would have hampered my healing, I think."

She's right. Depression hampers healing. Studies of people with certain cancers (breast, lymphoma, leukemia, and malignant melanoma) have found that treating their depression leads to increased survival. One study of people who were taught coping skills soon after being diagnosed with malignant melanoma showed a survival benefit extending into six years of follow-up.

Benefit Three: A Greater Sense of Well-Being

Other words for well-being are "happiness" or "contentment." It doesn't refer to a burst of delight, but a longstanding sense that life is full and complete. The authors of the *Handbook of Religion and Health* reviewed 100 research studies that looked at the connection between spirituality and well-being. "Of those studies, 79 reported at least one positive correlation between religious involvement and greater happiness, life satisfaction, morale, or positive affect [mood]."

When people consider themselves to have control over their lives, they tend to be happier. "In contrast, persons with no control over their lives—such as prisoners, nursing home patients, or the poverty stricken—have the least sense of well-being." People who believe God is caring for them have an enhanced sense of control, for if they are depending on God they can be less dependent on fellow humans or on mere chance.

> In many respects, an internalized, intrinsically motivated religious faith empowers the individual; prayer directed to an all-powerful and sympathetic God gives religious persons a tool that can be used to change their situation or acquire the strength to endure it.

Not being in control makes some people, like my husband Don, very uncomfortable. He likes to plan every detail of his day. But when I was diagnosed with cancer, a lot of what was happening to our family was out of his control.

"On one level it was difficult," he said, "but on another level it was a relief. Being in control is a tiresome process. I had to acknowledge that someone greater than me was in control—namely, God. Knowing that comforted me."

BENEFIT FOUR: LESS ANXIETY

Everyone has experienced anxiety. Most anxiety passes quickly, but when it engulfs people it can keep them from living normally. Research shows that "religion as a whole, especially intrinsic religiousness, tends to buffer against anxiety."

People with cancer who have a personal relationship with God are likely to see him as taking care of them, guiding them and their doctors to make the right decisions for their treatment. This leads to a greater sense of hope (that all will turn out well) and inner calm.

This can make a profound difference when life becomes difficult. Don and I went to a concert given by the singer Doug Oldham back when we were in medical school in Washington, D.C. He announced on stage that he had just been diagnosed with colon cancer. "I'm praying for healing," he said. "I believe God is able to heal me. But even if he doesn't, he is still God. And he is still good." Don and I were struck by how peaceful he was even though his life was threatened.

One study of a group of people who prayed for another group of people found that both groups had higher rates of self-esteem and lower rates of anxiety and depression at the end of the study. But the people doing the praying benefited even more than the people they were praying for.

BENEFIT FIVE: A MORE STABLE IMMUNE SYSTEM

My immune system is my key defense against tiny attacks on my body. Every day, thousands of bacteria and viruses that could have caused disease are destroyed by my immune system. It gobbles up stray cancer cells, too. I want my immune system to be as healthy as it can possibly be.

High levels of stress lead to greater production of substances (cortisol, catecholamines, interleukin-6) that hinder the immune system. Finding out I had cancer was stressful. Ironically, "the diagnosis of cancer itself may create psychological stress that then impairs the body's ability to contain the disease."

So how can I bolster my immune system? Researchers have studied this, also. Two ways: one—social support; two—religious involvement.

A number of studies show that signs of better immune system function increase as people have more emotional support and tangible social support. Friendships and close family relationships buffer people from the negative effects of stress.

Attending religious services leads to lower levels of interleukin-6 (IL-6), a blood protein that hampers people's immune systems. High levels of IL-6 are associated with various diseases, including certain kinds of cancer (B-cell lymphoma, multiple myeloma, head and neck cancer, and Hodgkin's disease). People who attended once a week or more had the lowest IL-6 levels, those who never attended had the highest levels, and intermediate attenders had intermediate levels.

> The relationship found between IL-6 and religious attendance suggests that persons who actively involve themselves in religious community may have more stable immune systems. It may also help explain why they have better physical health and longer survival.

A GOD WHO LOVES US

Even when people aren't part of a religious community, the community may reach out to them. Marcia G. found that to be true after she was diagnosed with breast cancer. "I'm not a religious person," she told me, "and I don't believe in God. But I'm amazed at the number of people who have stopped me to say, 'I'm praying for you.' When they do, I thank them.

"This has made me more respectful of others' beliefs and more appreciative of how their beliefs could be important to them. By saying 'I'm praying for you,' they're doing what they can to help. At one time that would have offended me, but now I'm a lot less cynical. I have more empathy with the idea that people would turn to God in times of trouble."

And indeed, people do turn to God in times of trouble. One study of 108 women with female cancers showed that one in two had become more religious since their diagnosis. "A very high 93 percent of the patients believed their religious lives helped them sustain their hopes." Not one became less religious.

But of course people can become less religious when faced with cancer. If they see God as someone who heals, always heals—and who indeed *must* heal them when they are sick—then their faith could be crushed if they are not healed. They could become angry. Either God was wrong to not heal them or their assumption about God was wrong.

Also, people may withdraw from a God they view negatively. That is, they are seeing him as someone who is punishing them with illness, who disapproves of them, or who doesn't care about what happens to them. One study looked at 577 hospitalized older adults—comparing those who saw God in a negative way with those who saw him in a positive way. When people saw God in a negative way they tended to have poorer physical health. They were also more likely to be depressed or have a worse quality of life compared to those who viewed God as someone who loved them and wanted a connection with them.

Another study then reported the follow-up of those hospitalized older adults. It looked at how many had died in the next two years. Those who had struggled with whether God loved them or cared about them had a 20-percent greater chance of being dead two years later.

Clearly it's not just believing in God that's important, but what exactly a person believes about who God is and how much he cares.

JUST HOW DEEP IS GOD'S LOVE?

Just three weeks after her wedding, 29-year-old Sara M. learned she had chronic myelogenous leukemia. But, significantly, just 12 months earlier she had "come back to God."

"Back then I believed there was a God," she said, "but not much else." Despite her diagnosis, she was convinced that God loved her and cared about her. God gave her strength, she believes, to face the grueling months of cancer treatments. She wonders how she could have faced it a year earlier, when her faith had been so much weaker. "Now I know God had been preparing me," she said.

Far from moving away from God since having cancer, she has actually drawn closer. "There's been a big growth spurt in my faith through this experience," she said.

The Christian scriptures are full of statements of God's love and care. David wrote in Psalm 34, "The LORD is close to the brokenhearted; he rescues those who are crushed in spirit." And in Psalm 145, "The LORD is kind and merciful, slow to get angry, full of unfailing love...The LORD is faithful in all he says; he is gracious in all he does. The LORD helps the fallen and lifts up those bent beneath their loads...The LORD is close to all who call on him, yes, to all who call on him sincerely."

And Jesus said, "Come to me, all of you who are weary and carry heavy burdens, and I will give you rest." Peter, who was one of Jesus' disciples, urged, "Give all your worries and cares to God, for he cares about what happens to you." And in Romans 8 Paul tells us that nothing can separate us from Christ's love:

> Death can't, and life can't. The angels can't, and the demons can't. Our fears for today, our worries about tomorrow, and even the powers of hell can't keep God's love away. Whether we are high above the sky or in the deepest ocean, nothing in all creation will ever be able to separate us from the love of God that is revealed in Christ Jesus our Lord.

WHAT ABOUT SUFFERING?

But what about when someone gets cancer? Does this prove that God's love didn't stretch far enough? Does suffering mean that God has removed his love?

Corrie ten Boom was a 50-year-old Christian woman in Holland who, along with her much-beloved sister and elderly father, hid Jewish people in her house during World War II. Arrested by the Nazis, Corrie suffered through her father's and sister's deaths and a brutal year in a concentration camp. Yet for the next 32 years, she shared with people all over the world that God is love. "There is no pit so deep that [God] is not deeper still."

Corrie ten Boom had an intrinsic spirituality. Her faith in God guided her life. Intrinsic, internalized faith leads to greater health, as research has shown. But more important even than health, it gives companionship—companionship with God himself.

When I was going through chemotherapy, I noticed that my oncologist, Dr. Marshall Leary, had a version of the following poem printed on the back of his appointment cards:

For cancer is so limited—
It cannot cripple love,
It cannot shatter hope,
It cannot corrode faith,
It cannot destroy peace,
It cannot kill friendship,
It cannot suppress memories,
It cannot silence courage,
It cannot invade the soul,
It cannot steal God's gift of eternal life,
It cannot quench the Holy Spirit,
It cannot lessen the power of the resurrection.

—Author unknown

I remember reading it over and over while sitting in his waiting room—usually with tears in my eyes. Cancer really is powerless. The worst it can do is touch my body. It has no authority over my emotions or my spirit.

If you have cancer...

Consider asking yourself these questions:

- Do I believe that "intrinsic" religion (religion that is the source of motivation) is more valuable than "extrinsic" religion (religion held in order to achieve certain goals)?

- Is my religion intrinsic or extrinsic? What steps can I take for it to become more intrinsic?

- What does God have to do with my cancer journey?

CHAPTER THIRTEEN

SEARCHING FOR MEANING

Three ways to find meaning ❧ *The greatest meaning*
Living with purpose ❧ *Looking forward to the good*

ANNE FRANK WAS A TEENAGER with adult-size problems. She was a Jewish schoolgirl in Holland when the Nazis overran her nation in World War II. In 1942, afraid for their lives, her family hid themselves in a cramped space they shared with others. Used to nonstop activity with friends and admirers, her heart heavy with the danger of their situation, Anne suffered. She poured out her feelings in her diary. Happily her diary survived the war. Sadly, she did not.

To read *Anne Frank: The Diary of a Young Girl* is to peek inside the mind of an insightful person—a person who develops from a typically self-absorbed 13-year-old into a 15-year-old striving to overcome her shortcomings. After 20 months in hiding, Anne looked back at her carefree life of "before" and asked, "What is left of this girl?" She'd like to once again live the life of "before"—but only for a week.

> At the end of that week, I...would be only too thankful to listen to anyone who began to talk about something sensible. I don't want followers, but friends, admirers who fall not for a flattering smile but for what one does and for one's character.

She realized that "the Anne of 1944" was far superior to "the Anne of 1942," though the transformation had cost her much suffering. She was giving her ordeal purpose and value—it had made her a better person. And so her pain withered and her hope flourished.

DOES LIFE HAVE MEANING?

Victor Frankl, a doctor of psychiatry who held that people can cope with any situation as long as they can apply meaning to it, would have approved. He'd have approved back then, that is, if he could have met Anne Frank. But he couldn't, for he was fighting his own battle for survival at the time—in the Nazi concentration camp at Auschwitz.

The three years he spent there—and in three other death camps—overflowed with extreme suffering. He wrote about the truths he learned in *Man's Search for Meaning*, which was first published a year after he was liberated.

While a prisoner, he expected he'd die in the camps. Yet he determined to try to make some sense of his death. He observed that "the prisoner who had lost faith in the future—his future—was doomed." He wrote of several men whose plunge into despair was followed quickly by death.

One day when "the endless little problems of our miserable life" were drowning him, he had a moment of revelation. He saw himself in a warm and well-lit lecture hall "giving a lecture on the psychology of the concentration camp" to "an attentive audience on comfortable upholstered seats." His present troubles shrank and seemed as though they were already a part of his past.

He'd succeeded in "rising above the situation" and seeing his suffering in the context of the rest of his life. And so he increased the possibility he'd have a "rest of his life." For at that moment suffering lost its power over him. "Emotion, which is suffering, ceases to be suffering as soon as we form a clear and precise picture of it."

Frankl fulfilled the vision of that day in the concentration camp—yes, a thousand times over. Until his death in 1997 he lectured worldwide on the system of thought he had pioneered: that a person's deepest desire is for life to have meaning.

When people suffer, this deep desire rises to the surface. They can find meaning in their suffering—and in a broader sense, their life—in many ways. These ways, according to Frankl, can be placed in three broad categories:

1. *Creating a work or doing a deed:* that is, leaving a legacy by some tangible action

2. *Experiencing something or encountering someone:* that is, seeing something long anticipated, or growing in one's love for a highly valued person

3. *Facing the inevitable suffering with dignity:* that is, when suffering is unavoidable, accepting it and so being elevated to a position of worth

1. Creating a Work or Doing a Deed

When John Hill was diagnosed with prostate cancer in August 2000, he was a newspaper journalist. But even the wild world of Louisiana politics didn't interest him at that time—he could think only of cancer. So he chose to write about his diagnosis and his cancer journey in a series of articles. "I wrote what was on my mind: 'It's malignant' is where I started. I felt compelled to get as many men as possible to have the prostate cancer screenings."

He succeeded. Six weeks later, during Prostate Cancer Awareness Week, 1600 men made appointments for free screenings at LSU Health Sciences Center in Shreveport—up from 1000 the year before. Many said they were there because they'd read his articles.

> Once more I was humbled by the power of the press. This diary, my story of my journey with prostate cancer, has had an immediate and measurable impact.
>
> One [editor] told me that I sounded more like myself than I have in more than a month. It was because for the first time in my journalistic career, I felt I have made a real, tangible contribution.
>
> I made a difference by my decision to discuss the disease and its impact on me publicly.

To bring meaning, an achievement need not impact as many people as John Hill's. At first, it may impact only one—the person who suffers.

Benjamin Lawrence was a sailor aboard the whaling ship *Essex* when a whale broke apart the ship and the crew was cast adrift in open boats with scant supplies. Few of them survived the 93 days on the open sea. Two who did were Owen Chase, who kept a journal, and Lawrence, who twisted stray strands of rope into a small coil of twine. Having a task kept each of them from losing hope and probably kept them alive.

2. Experiencing Something or Encountering Someone

In 1990, Renee B. nearly died from childbirth complications, and afterward she went through a difficult, multiyear recovery period. "I'm grateful for the love my family and my friends showed me," she says. "Their love was unconditional. They didn't say, 'You've been sick long enough.' No, they kept bringing me meals and kept caring for my children and kept doing the things I didn't have the energy to do. What they did allowed me to 'sit back' and get well."

Receiving such love humbled Renee, and it cemented those relationships. She realized she owed these people a debt she could never repay. "But what I've carried away from my illness is that the debt I owe is not so much to my family and friends—for they are healthy, and I pray they stay that way—but to others who need my help, even if it's only something small." Her fellow human beings are worthy of her service.

Renee also made great leaps in her relationship with God through her years of weakness. "Just before I got sick I had been in a group that was studying Philippians 4:13: 'I can do all things through Christ which strengtheneth me.' That verse got me through the most dangerous time in the beginning. I'd say it over and over, even though I couldn't get out of bed at the time.

"Then when I faced such a long recovery—with infections, terrible treatments, and the emotional pain of not being able to have more children—I realized how much I needed God and also that I wasn't 'the master of my own destiny.' He's all I have, but he's enough. He's more than enough." Renee sees value in her time of suffering, for it allowed her to grow in her love for people and for God.

At age 34, Debbie has never had a life-threatening illness, but she suffered through a turbulent and harsh childhood. She knows the misery she felt as a teenager helped push her toward God. She has found his love to be completely satisfying. "I wouldn't exchange what I know about God in order to have a different past," she says.

3. Facing Inevitable Suffering with Dignity

Victor Frankl considered this third way to find meaning in life to be the most important one of all. He knew that all people will suffer, provided they live long enough. They can choose their response to that suffering.

"There are situations," Frankl wrote, "in which one is cut off from the opportunity to do one's work or to enjoy one's life; but what never can be ruled out is the unavoid-ability of suffering. In accepting this challenge to suffer bravely, life has a meaning up to the last moment, and it retains this meaning literally to the end."

Our society is so quick to equate meaning with useful-ness, but we are too limited in our understanding. People who are created by God have value—and their lives have meaning regardless of whether they are useful.

In *The Faith Factor*, a book that links religious faith and practices with better physical health, Dr. Dale Matthews tells the story of one of his patients. Melanie had once owned a retail store and had been active in her church. Now she had chronic fatigue syndrome and could barely get out of bed in the morning. Just washing her hair exhausted her. She grieved the loss of her former life.

Dr. Matthews suggested she pray. "You can pray, for yourself and for other people, even when you're at your worst physically." She welcomed this idea and reported back that she once again felt fulfilled. "Having a prayer ministry," he wrote, "gives her a sense of purpose and satisfaction that was lacking in her life because of her disabling illness."

I also believe that her praying was "doing something," because prayer leads to real results. So in that sense Melanie was also gaining meaning by "creating a work or doing a deed." But by choosing to pray she was also transforming her suffering and herself at the same time. She couldn't give herself more energy, but she wasn't powerless, either. Infusing her suffering with meaning allowed her to cope with it.

SUPERMEANING AND A SUPERBEING

Victor Frankl spoke of another meaning that went beyond *creating a work or doing a deed, experiencing some-thing or encountering someone*, or *facing inevitable suffering with dignity*. It is a meaning that arches over these three ways to finding meaning. He called it "a Supermeaning, a meaning so comprehensive that you can no longer grasp it....And a religious person may identify Supermeaning as something paralleling a Superbeing, and this Superbeing we would call God."

Long ago Thomas Aquinas observed, "There is within every soul a thirst for happiness and meaning." In the 700 years since those words were written they've been proved true countless times. Neither money nor fame satisfies the thirst he talks about. Michael Jordan, the basketball superstar, has had plenty of both, yet in his biographical IMAX movie he echoes Aquinas. "I believe we're here on this earth for a purpose," he said. "And we don't know when that time will be over. We need to appreciate the time we have."

I myself also believe "we're here on this earth for a purpose." When I was diagnosed with Hodgkin's lymphoma, I couldn't imagine how my having cancer fit into that purpose. I struggled to understand. I asked God for help, and over time he gave me snatches of insight: I'd have more compassion for my patients because I, too, had been sick. My impact would be greater because suffering people listen more willingly to someone who has also suffered. And I could write about my experiences and thus reach out to many I'd never meet in person.

These snatches helped to give me hope. But there was an even bigger insight that helped the most. It came from seeing myself as God's child—God's much-loved child. And since he is a good father—unlike so many human fathers—this thing wouldn't be happening to me if it wasn't somehow for my good. I might not understand it then, and I may never understand it, but I have a hope for the future that goes beyond this life on earth.

The apostle Paul put it this way: "Since we are his children, we will share his treasures—for everything God gives to his Son, Christ, is ours, too. But if we are to share his glory, we must also share his suffering. Yet what we suffer now is nothing compared to the glory he will give us later."

ACTIVE COPING

In *The Story of Eric Liddell,* a biographical videotape of the 1924 Olympic gold-medal-winning runner, a woman who knew him said something remarkable. Kari Malcolm had been in a mission school in China when the Japanese placed her and a few thousand other Europeans—including Liddell—in Weihsien Camp for the remainder of World War II. As a teenager separated from her parents, she felt as if her life had ended. The locks on the prison gates kept her inside the camp, and her hopes and dreams outside:

> I had planned to go to college at age 17, but instead I went to prison. But the Lord worked in me to show me he had other plans and this was part of it. I came to the place where I said, "Lord, I am willing to stay in this prison for the rest of my life if I can only know you." And at that point I was free! It was as if the gates had been opened. I was released in my spirit.

Kari's relationship with God was an active one, not a passive one. Many cancer patients interact with God in a similar manner. Medical research is starting to see the positive benefits of this way of coping with suffering. A 1999 article in a medical journal said, "This interactive relationship [with God] provides patients with a sense of connection and involvement rather than isolation, helplessness and hopelessness." Connecting with God helps people cope.

That same article states,

> Religious convictions may help to give the illness experience meaning and perspective. Such a cognitive coping style has been associated in other

studies with lower levels of anxiety, as well as greater activity and flexibility in dealing with illness.

Living Life Forward

Even before I had cancer, I remember hearing about survivors who said they were "glad they'd had cancer." How could they say that? Then when I was diagnosed, such a statement seemed even more inconceivable. The months of treatment were so miserable I couldn't imagine ever being glad they had happened. But now I'm starting to understand.

Since I was diagnosed with cancer, I've definitely grown as a person—developing qualities that benefit me. I've reflected on how I've spent my time in the past and how I should spend it in the future. My time on earth, I learned, is not limitless. I've chosen to do some things "now" that I might have otherwise put off. People and experiences that I would previously have taken for granted are more precious to me now. I'm not glad to have had cancer, but I am glad for what I've gained through the experience.

My husband, Don, isn't glad that I had cancer either, but like me he sees value in it. "The experience was hard, but the fruit is priceless," he said. "For me, the things that were really important came into sharp focus."

"Smooth seas do not make skillful sailors," goes the African proverb. I think this is true—and I do want to become a skillful sailor—but given a choice I'd still choose smooth seas. I don't like to suffer, but I have to keep reminding myself that it's the only way to become a skillful sailor. God will be with me in the roughest seas and through the fiercest gales.

Don and I both have a sense that God is using the difficult times of our lives to produce something good. I think this is what James meant when he wrote in the Bible,

Dear brothers and sisters, whenever trouble comes your way, let it be an opportunity for joy. For when your faith is tested, your endurance has a chance to grow. So let it grow, for when your endurance is fully developed, you will be strong in character and ready for anything.

I want to be strong in character and ready for anything—even if I have to go through trouble to get that way.

Soren Kierkegaard, a great thinker of the nineteenth century, noted, "Life can only be understood backwards, but it must be lived forwards." He wasn't saying that I will always perfectly understand life when I look back—and I don't—but that my best chance at understanding will come from looking backward. Looking forward, I may not have complete control over everything that happens to me, but I do have control over how I respond to those things.

When I look back, I see the difficult experiences of my life helping to strengthen my character and draw me closer to God. Knowing that this has been true in the past gives me confidence that it will also be true in the future.

If you have cancer...

Consider asking yourself these questions:

- How does my having cancer fit in the context of "the rest of my life"?

- Victor Frankl offered three possible ways to find meaning in suffering:

  creating a work or doing a deed

  experiencing something or encountering someone

  facing inevitable suffering with dignity

  Which of these might apply to me? Is there anything that I can do—or any way that I can grow—that would not have been possible if I had not had cancer?

- Am I able to see my present troubles as a way to strengthen my character and make me ready for anything? Am I growing closer to God?

AFTERWORD

❧

WHATEVER THE REASON YOU HAVE read this book—whether you are someone with cancer, a family member or friend of someone with cancer, or a person interested in the way medical care happens—I wish you well. I want this book to point you toward the answers to any questions you have been asking. But for those of you who have recently received a cancer diagnosis, I have some special words.

I hope this book has helped you understand some of the things you are going through and has helped you prepare for some of the things you will be going through in the coming weeks and months. I, too, once stood on the edge of the gaping chasm, taking my first step onto the bridge that is the cancer journey. The bridge may look rickety, but it has supported millions of travelers before you and will support many millions more.

And here's the good news: That bridge is getting stronger. Every year cancer researchers find new ways to successfully treat cancer. And they're not just finding more effective drugs that tackle cancer "from the outside in"—now they're starting to treat cancer "from the inside out."

Cancer researchers are using newfound knowledge of genes—the genes that are inside cells and cause them to act the way they do. Learning the secrets of the inner workings of cells means that cancer researchers can start changing the way those cells behave. It's as if, for many years, people treating cancer have been fishing with nets and—until recently—have focused only on weaving bigger and finer nets. Now they're learning how to make "smart nets"—nets that know exactly where the fish are and are able to seek them out and capture them.

So am I saying this is a good time to have cancer? In the sense that it's never a good time to have a life-threatening illness, the answer is *no*. But in the sense that people's cancers are now responding to groundbreaking treatments that were unknown a few years ago, the answer is *yes*.

So be encouraged! And as you step out onto your bridge back to health—your cancer journey—may you walk with God by your side. My wish for you is that someday you will be able to look back and, despite the difficulties and challenges, see that your journey has helped you grow into more of the person God intended for you to be when you were born. I think the apostle Paul was touching on a great mystery when he wrote in the Bible that he was rejoicing in his sufferings—which were many, by the way—"because we know that suffering produces perseverance; perseverance, character; and character, hope. And hope does not disappoint us, because God has poured out his love into our hearts by the Holy Spirit, whom he has given us."

Do I understand all this? No—I've caught just a glimpse. But I know my experience with cancer has developed my perseverance, my character, and my hope.

"A clay pot sitting in the sun will always be a clay pot. It has to go through the white heat of the furnace to become porcelain." May this time of suffering become something beautiful in your life also.

—Amy Givler
www.amygivler.com

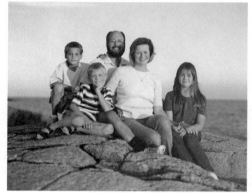

The Givler family, 2001
Left to right: Pete (10), John (8),
Don and Amy, Martha Grace (11)

A Guide to Medical Resources

Cancer-Related Web Sites
Cancer-Related Books
Articles in Medical Journals
Medical Libraries

Cancer-Related Web Sites

Evaluating Web Sites

There are far more Web sites with useful cancer information than I can list. Therefore I've limited myself to just a few well-maintained and reliable sites that I would have wanted to have had access to when I was first diagnosed (the listing starts on page 195).

As a disclaimer, I couldn't possibly have evaluated all the information contained in all these Web sites. Also, the information changes frequently. But I've tried to pick Web sites that offer a solid medical perspective, sensitivity to the emotional needs of readers, and information that's easy to understand—and use.

All of these Web sites also have links to other Web sites. How can you evaluate those other Web sites? Here are some tips:

- The site should state clearly who runs it and what its purpose is. After all, it costs money to run a Web site—so who is spending that money, and why? You'll see

I've chosen several government Web sites. I understand the government's viewpoint—it wants its citizens healthy, and it isn't trying to sell anything. And besides, it's paying for the Web site with my tax dollars. In that sense I've already paid for the information.

* Any sponsorship or funding by commercial interests should be clearly identified.

* The information should be regularly updated, and it should be based on medical research. The best sites have an editorial board whose members are well-qualified to review the information for accuracy.

* You should be able to contact the Web master or organization for questions or feedback.

* The National Cancer Institute's Web site has an excellent guide to evaluating other medical Web sites. Go to <www.cancer.gov/CancerInformation/ otherwebsites> and then click on "10 Things to Know About Evaluating Medical Resources on the Web."

Web Site Warning

And what should you be wary of? People with cancer are at risk of being drawn into buying questionable products. Their lives are being threatened, and they may be vulnerable to false promises.

* Beware if a drug or treatment is available from only one source, for only a limited time.

* Beware if the Web site is peppered with phrases such as "scientific breakthrough," "miraculous cure," "exclusive product," "secret formula," and "ancient ingredient."

- Beware if the Web site prominently features case histories from customers claiming amazing cures.

- Beware if the product claims to cure or treat dozens of widely varying symptoms.

- Beware if the Web site claims that the government, the medical profession, or research scientists have conspired to suppress the product they're selling.

Useful Web Sites (Listed Alphabetically)

Association of Online Cancer Resources
<www.acor.org>
ACOR is a nonprofit organization that was created to provide support for people touched by cancer. At its heart is a collection of online communities—hundreds of mailing lists that allow participants to share information and give each other support. ACOR also hosts Web sites with cancer information, information provided by many different individuals and groups. There are resource guides and links to recent research.

American Cancer Society
<www.cancer.org>
The ACS is a nonprofit organization that provides information and tangible help for people with cancer. Calling them (1-800-227-2345) will also connect you to your local division of the ACS. They can give help in locating financial and practical resources, also.

CancerBACUP
<www.cancerbacup.org.uk>
CancerBACUP is the United Kingdom's leading cancer-information service, and it is indeed packed with information—more than 3000 pages. The information is practical and up-to-date. I found the entire Web site to be very readable and easy to navigate.

Cancer Care

<www.cancercare.org>

Cancer Care is a nonprofit organization that provides emotional support, information, and practical help to people with cancer and their loved ones. It's a national social-service agency that offers telephone support, online support groups, limited funds for transportation, and much more. The Web site is well-designed and full of information.

ClinicalTrials.gov

<www.clinicaltrials.gov>

This site is maintained by the National Institutes of Health (NIH). Through it, people can quickly search for clinical studies sponsored by the NIH, other U.S. agencies, and the pharmaceutical industry. It includes more than 6000 clinical trials in nearly 70,000 locations worldwide.

Healthfinder

<www.healthfinder>

Healthfinder was developed by the U.S. Department of Health and Human Services to provide links to reliable health information on the web. The actual information is on other Web sites. HHS has carefully reviewed the health information in thousands of sites. Included on this Web site are links to more than 1800 government agencies, nonprofit organizations, and universities.

HealthWeb

<www.healthweb.org>

This is a site sponsored by a group of medical libraries in the Midwest. It provides links to hundreds of other health-information sites on the Internet.

Major Cancer Centers

The National Cancer Institute (NCI) keeps a list of the "NCI-designated cancer centers," with their contact information, at <www.cancer.gov/cancercenters/centerslist.html>.

Updated regularly, as of this writing the list includes 60 centers in 32 states. I describe NCI-designated cancer centers in chapter 7.

Many cancer centers maintain well-run Web sites with excellent information. Of course, each cancer center wants you to decide to go there, but the contents of these sites will be helpful whether or not you decide to go. To give you a flavor of such Web sites, here are the addresses of the sites of what most people consider the two top cancer treatment centers:

* *Memorial Sloan–Kettering Cancer Center* (in New York City)
  <www.MSKCC.org>

* *M.D. Anderson Cancer Center* (affiliated with the University of Texas in Houston)
  <www.mdanderson.org>

MEDLINEplus Health Information
<www.medlineplus.gov>
Maintained for the health consumer by the U.S. National Library of Medicine (cancer is one of hundreds of health topics on this site), MEDLINEplus provides links to thousands of other medically related Web sites. It also contains current health news, information about generic and brand-name drugs, online medical dictionaries, directories of doctors, dentists, and hospitals, and much, much more.

National Cancer Institute
<www.cancer.gov>
This is a massive site with solid cancer information. It's an excellent place to explore first. The National Cancer Institute (NCI) is the U.S. government's agency for cancer research and training. Happily, its mission also includes sharing cancer information with the public, and this Web site flows from that mission.

People can also call NCI (1-800-4-CANCER) to receive its publications. They can also view those publications on the Web site or can order up to 20 from the Web site to be mailed to them for free. These are called "Cancer Information Summaries." Once you're at <www.cancer.gov>, click on "Cancer Information," then "PDQ" (which stands for "Physician Data Query"), then "PDQ Cancer Information Summaries: Treatment" to see a list of all the summaries. You can choose to read the material intended for "patients" or that for "health professionals." The advantage of the material for "health professionals" is that it has references to many medical journal articles.

Dozens of other "Cancer Information Summaries" are listed under the categories "Complementary and Alternative Medicine," "Screening/Detection," "Prevention," "Genetics," and "Supportive Care."

OncoLink
<www.oncolink.com>
Sponsored by the University of Pennsylvania Cancer Center, OncoLink provides cancer news (updated daily) and easy-to-understand cancer information for patients and their families, as well as for medical professionals. It also has a large gallery of art created by people touched by cancer. There are reviews of cancer books and videos and a list of peer-reviewed journals with links to the journals' Web sites.

Patient-Centered Guides
<www.patientcenters.com>
Patient-Centered Guides are books you can purchase, but this organization also has extensive excerpts from the guides on their Web site. These books were written by people who have been touched by the condition they are writing about. They're very readable and contain stories of real people, and yet they are careful to include well-researched

medical information. The site describes the guides as "a mix of medical, practical and emotional information, grounded in Western medicine, told by people who have been there."

CANCER-RELATED BOOKS

An extensive list of cancer-related books is given on the Association of Cancer Online Resource's Web site (<www.acor.org/biblio>). The list is broken down into 16 sections and has more than 100 titles, along with a short description of each.

Of those many books, the following (listed alphabetically) are the ones I most wish had existed when I was diagnosed:

1. *The Complete Cancer Survival Guide: Everything You Must Know and Where to Go for State-of-the-Art Treatment of the 25 Most Common Forms of Cancer*
   Peter Teeley and Philip Bashe
   Random House, Inc.
   972 pages, April 2000
   List price*: $19.95

   This is not only a comprehensive book that covers the 25 most common cancers well, but it is also interspersed with stories of Peter Teeley's personal experience with colon cancer and interviews with top cancer doctors. It's well-organized, and the writing is clear.

2. *Diagnosis Cancer: Your Guide Through the First Few Months (revised edition)*
   Wendy S. Harpham, M.D.
   W.W. Norton & Company, Inc.
   192 pages, November 1997
   List price: $13.00

---

* List prices are as of mid-2002.

Dr. Harpham wrote the first edition of her book soon after completing chemotherapy for lymphoma. Using a question-and-answer format, she covers an extensive list of topics that a person new to the world of medicine might want to know about.

3. *Everyone's Guide to Cancer Therapy: How Cancer is Diagnosed, Treated, and Managed Day to Day (3rd edition)*
Malin Dollinger, M.D., Ernest H. Rosenbaum, M.D., and Greg Cable
Andrews McMeel Publishing
848 pages, January 1998
List price: $21.95

This book is packed with sophisticated cancer treatment information yet is written in plain English. One section addresses the emotional needs of people with cancer, and another addresses new advances in cancer research. Another section describes specific cancers—their diagnosis, their treatment, and their follow-up. It suggests questions to ask doctors, and it has an extensive list of resources in the back.

4. *The Human Side of Cancer: Living with Hope, Coping with Uncertainty*
Jimmie C. Holland, M.D., and Sheldon Lewis
HarperCollins Publishers Inc.
368 pages, October 2001
List price: $14.00

Because of her 23 years helping people with cancer cope at one of the country's top cancer centers (Memorial Sloan–Kettering in New York City), Dr. Holland understands the emotions of the cancer journey. This book brings her knowledge and experience both to those who cope with stressful situations by being assertive and to those who are more reserved. Family members and friends who want to understand how their loved one is responding to his or her diagnosis will particularly benefit by reading this book.

ARTICLES IN MEDICAL JOURNALS

In the Notes (beginning on page 205), I've included the full references for the medical journal articles I've referred to, in case you would like to look them up for yourself. "But how," you may be asking, "do I do that?"

The National Library of Medicine has a short summary of almost every important medical journal article (called an "abstract") listed on its Web site. Here's how to reach those abstracts:

1. Go to <www.nlm.nih.gov>.

2. Click on "Health Information" (first on list).

3. Then click on "MEDLINE/PubMed" (second on list).

4. Look on the left-hand side of the screen for "Single Citation Matcher," which is under the "PubMed Services" heading. Click on it.

5. The form you next see does not need to be completely filled out. I'd suggest just putting in the "Journal Name," the "Volume Number," and the "Issue Number," and the last name of the author (you don't need to add the author's initials as it suggests). Filling in the "Date," "First Page," and "Title Words" is unnecessary. Then click "Search."

6. When the reference to the article comes up, click on it. Then you will see the abstract.

7. Sometimes the search won't work. If it's any comfort, it doesn't always work for me either. Everything has to be spelled perfectly. What I do if this process doesn't work is type in only the journal name, the volume number, and the issue number. Then I get a list of all the articles in that issue—typically around 20. I scroll down until I see the article I'm looking for.

The National Library of Medicine provides only abstracts of articles, but that may be all you want to read. If you'd like the full text of an article, it may be available for free through the medical journal's Web site. On the page with the abstract of the article you want to read, there's usually a button that links you to the medical journal's Web site. The journal may ask you to pay a fee before you can read the full article, though—and those fees can quickly add up.

An added benefit to having the full article is having the references to other, related articles at the end of the article you're looking at.

So you may want to get in your car and go to a…

MEDICAL LIBRARY

Medical libraries are found in every medical school and in almost all of the larger hospitals. The bigger the medical library, the more journals it will subscribe to. Most medical libraries allow some public access—it helps especially if you call first and let the librarian know what you are interested in.

If the library doesn't subscribe to the journal that contains the article you want, then the librarian can order the article—again, for a fee. That fee may or may not be less than what the journal's Web site asks for access to the article.

If you're looking for only one or two articles, you may be able to ask the librarian to get them for you with a simple phone call.

All medical librarians I've ever worked with have been excellent at what they do and eager to get information into the hands of someone it will benefit. For a link to more than 130 of the larger medical libraries, go to <www.nlm.nih.gov/medlineplus/libraries.html>.

NOTES

&

To the reader—Citations from journals are noted in this format: Author(s), article name, journal name, volume number, issue number (date, if given): page reference.

For example:
Wendy Harpham, M.D., "Raising the Curtain on Cancer," *Postgraduate Medicine* 102, no. 3 (September 1997): p. 242.

Chapter 1—Looking at Cancer in a New Way

Page 15: There are more than eight...
Maria Hewitt and Joseph V. Simone, eds., *Ensuring Quality Cancer Care* (Washington, D.C.: National Academy Press, 1999), p. 13.

Page 15: Only 1.3 million...; In the 1950s only 35...
Ahmedin Jemal, DVM, PhD, et al, "Cancer Statistics 2002," *CA: A Cancer Journal for Clinicians* 52, no. 1 (January/February 2002): p. 42.

Page 16: "None of the basic..."
Wendy Harpham, M.D., "Raising the Curtain on Cancer," *Postgraduate Medicine* 102, no. 3 (September 1997): p. 242.

Page 18: "Even though I walk..."
Psalm 23:4.

Chapter 2—Hearing—or *Not* Hearing—the Word "Cancer" for the First Time

Page 22: "With good luck..."
Rudyard Kipling, *Captains Courageous* (New York: Amsco School Publications, Inc.), p. 12.

Page 23: "The general feeling..."
Donald Oken, M.D., "What to Tell Cancer Patients," *Journal of the American Medical Association* 175, no. 13 (April 1, 1961): p. 92.

Page 25: "The worst fear..."
Robert Buckman, "Breaking Bad News: Why Is It Still So Difficult?" *British Medical Journal* 288 (May 26, 1984): p. 1597.

Page 25: "We're seldom angry..."
Cecil Murphey, *Simply Living* (Louisville, KY: Westminster John Knox Press, 2001), p. 111.

Page 26: "A soft answer..."
Proverbs 15:1 RSV.

Page 26: "laymen either do not..."
ranz Ingelfinger, M.D., "Arrogance," *New England Journal of Medicine* 303, no. 26 (December 25, 1980): pp. 1507-1511.

Page 26: One research study...
M. Omne-Ponten, et al, "Psychosocial Adjustment Among Women with Breast Cancer Stages I and II: Six-Year Follow-Up of Consecutive Patients," *Journal of Clinical Oncology* 12, no. 9 (September 1994): pp. 1778-1782.

Page 27: "Not knowing about..."
Barrie R. Cassileth, Ph.D., et.al, "Information and Participation Preferences Among Cancer Patients," *Annals of Internal Medicine* 92 (1980): p. 835.

Page 27: "Clinicians often..."
Cassileth, p. 835.

Page 27: Hoping for freedom...
Aaron Sardell, Psy.D., and Steven Trierweiler, Ph.D., "Disclosing the Cancer Diagnosis," *Cancer* (December 1, 1993): p. 3364.

Page 29: "Be not angry..."
Mark Water, compiler, *The New Encyclopedia of Christian Quotations* (Grand Rapids, MI: Baker Books, 2000), p. 50.

Page 29: "Someone once said..."
Frederica Mathewes-Green, "Unrighteous Indignation," *Christianity Today,* October 23, 2000, p. 117.

Chapter 3—Adjusting Emotionally to the Diagnosis

Page 31: "Gandalf came by"; "Sorry! I don't..."
J.R.R. Tolkien, *The Hobbit* (New York: Ballantine Books, 1937, 1966), pp. 17,19.

Page 37: "God has so made..."
Granger Westberg, *Good Grief* (Philadelphia: Fortress Press, 1962, 1971), pp. 21,23.

Page 39: "O LORD, hear me..."
Psalm 5:1-2 NLT.

Page 39: "I cried out..."
Psalm 30:8-10 NLT.

Page 40: "It is important..."
Jimmie Holland, M.D., and Sheldon Lewis, *The Human Side of Cancer* (New York: HarperCollins Publishers Inc., 2000), pp. 45-46.

Page 42: "We finally begin..."
Westberg, p. 61.

Page 44: "My dear Bilbo!"
Tolkien, p. 284.

Chapter 4—Entering the Medical World

Page 49: "Setting foot..."
Peter Teeley and Philip Bashe, *The Complete Cancer Survival Guide* (New York: Bantam Doubleday Dell Publishing Group, 2000), p. 315.

Page 50: "Our fear of death..."; "If we get well..."
Alice Stewart Trillin, "Of Dragons and Garden Peas; A Cancer Patient Talks to Doctors," *New England Journal of Medicine* 304 (1981): pp. 699, 700.

Page 53: "Medical education..."
Michael Simpson, et al, "Doctor-Patient Communication: The Toronto Consensus Statement," *British Medical Journal* 303 (1991): p. 1386.

Page 53: "To cover the vast..."
William Bennett Bean, ed., *Sir William Osler: Aphorisms from His Bedside Teachings and Writings,* collected by Robert Bennett Bean (Springfield, IL: Charles C. Thomas, 1968), p. 40.

Page 54: "Care more particularly..."
Bean, ed., p. 97.

Page 54: In the same speech...
Franz Ingelfinger, "Arrogance," *New England Journal of Medicine* 303 (1980): pp.1507-1511.

Page 55: "Doctors for various..."
Ingelfinger, p. 1510.

Chapter 5—How Medical Care Becomes Trustworthy

Page 59: "shrugged their shoulders..."
Irving Robbin, *Giants of Medicine* (New York: Grosset & Dunlap, Inc., 1962), p. 57.

Page 65: "The litigation experience..."
Robyn Shapiro, et al, "A Survey of Sued and Nonsued Physicians and Suing Patients," *Archives of Internal Medicine* 149 (1989): p. 2196.

Pages 66-67: "Family, Friends..."; "The lure of..."
Wendy Harpham, "Alternative Therapies for Curing Cancer: What Do Patients Want? What Do Patients Need?" *CA: A Cancer Journal for Clinicians* 51 (2001): pp. 132, 133.

Page 67: "Many forms of..."
As cited in Gary Stewart, D.Min., et al, *Basic Questions on Alternative Medicine* (Grand Rapids, MI: Kregel Publications, 1998), p. 22.

Page 68: "Reflecting on..."
Jimmie Holland, M.D., and Sheldon Lewis, *The Human Side of Cancer* (New York: HarperCollins Publishers Inc., 2000), p. 52.

Chapter 6—Choosing a Healthy Attitude

Page 72: "Why did you do..."
E.B. White, *Charlotte's Web* (New York: Harper & Brothers Publishers, 1952), p. 164.

Page 72: "Lord, do not hold..."
Acts 7:60.

Page 75: In 1979 a British researcher...
S. Greer, et al, "Psychological Response to Breast Cancer: Effect on Outcome," *The Lancet* (October 13, 1979): pp. 785-787.

Page 77: "Over the years..."
Jimmie Holland, M.D., and Sheldon Lewis, *The Human Side of Cancer* (New York: HarperCollins Publishers Inc., 2000), p. 28.

Page 77: One large study...
Maggie Watson, et al, "Influence of Psychological Response on Survival in Breast Cancer: A Population-Based Cohort Study," *The Lancet* (October 16, 1999): p. 1335.

Page 79: "The opposite of hope..."
Holland, p. 265.

Page 83: "the witnesses laid..."
Acts 7:58.

Page 83: "The Church owes..."
Quoted in William Barclay, *The Acts of the Apostles,* rev. ed., (Philadelphia: The Westminster Press, 1976), p. 62.

Chapter 7—Thinking Through the Options Promptly

Page 90: "Oncologists today..."
Jimmie C. Holland, M.D., and Sheldon Lewis, *The Human Side of Cancer* (New York: HarperCollins Publishers Inc., 2000), p. 62.

Page 92: The number of cancer doctors...
Maria Hewitt and Joseph V. Simone, eds., *Ensuring Quality Cancer Care* (Washington, D.C.: National Academy Press, 1999), p. 26.

Page 92: "In Italy..."
Andrea Piga, et al, "Attitudes of Non-Oncology Physicians Dealing with Cancer Patients: A Survey Based on Clinical Scenarios in Ancona Province, Central Italy," *Tumori* 82 (1996): p. 423.

Page 94: But Bruce Hillner...
Bruce E. Hillner, M.D., "Is Cancer Care Best at High-Volume Providers?" *Current Oncology Reports* 3 (2001): p. 408.

Page 94: In *The Complete*...
Peter Teeley and Philip Bashe, *The Complete Cancer Survival Guide* (New York: Bantam Doubleday Dell Publishing Group, Inc., 2000), pp. 293-298.

Chapter 8—Getting Specialized Help

Page 103: "Follow me"
Matthew 9:9.

Page 105: "I'm stunned by..."
Carol Krucoff, "A Scary Diagnosis," *Prevention,* July 2001, p. 134.

Page 107: "A significant lag..."
Leslie Ford, et al, "Diffusion and Adoption of State-of-the-Art Therapy," *Seminars in Oncology* 17, no. 4 (August, 1990): p. 485.

Page 108: Often, people end up..."
Maria Hewitt and Joseph V. Simone, eds., *Ensuring Quality Cancer Care* (Washington, D.C.: National Academy Press, 1999), pp. 117-118.

Page 108: "Where organizational factors..."
Bruce E. Hillner, M.D., et al, "Hospital and Physician Volume, or Specialization and Outcomes in Cancer Treatment," *Journal of Clinical Oncology* 18, no. 11 (June 2000): p. 2336.

Pages 108-109: In the report...; This report also describes...; "Ensure that patients undergoing..."
Hewitt and Simone, pp. 119-125; 125,126,127; 217.

Page 112: "The process is..."
John N. Lukens, M.D., "Progress Resulting from Clinical Trials: Solid Tumors in Childhood Cancer," *Cancer* supplement 74, no. 9 (November 1, 1994): p. 2710.

Page 112: Among younger adults...
National Cancer Institute Web site, accessed 6/10/02: <www.cancer.gov/clinical_trials>.

Page 112: A study of children...
Sharon Murphy, M.D., "The National Impact of Clinical Cooperative Group Trials for Pediatric Cancer," *Medical and Pediatric Oncology* 24 (1995): pp. 279-280.

Page 113: "Phase III trials..."
Jimmie C. Holland, M.D., and Sheldon Lewis, *The Human Side of Cancer* (New York: HarperCollins Publishers Inc., 2000), p. 113.

Page 114: This research shows..."
J.J. Guidry, et al, "Cost Considerations as Potential Barriers to Cancer Treatment," *Cancer Practice* 6, no. 3 (May/June 1998): pp. 182-187.

Page 114: "Patients, particularly minorities..."
J.J. Guidry, et al, "Transportation as a Barrier to Cancer Treatment," *Cancer Practice* 5, no. 6 (November/December 1997): pp. 361-366.

Page 114: Also, people older than...
Hewitt and Simone, pp. 60-61.

Chapter 9—Making Decisions in Partnership

Page 120: "The man who has..."
Saint Augustine, *The Confessions,* vol. 4, number 4, p. 399.

Page 121: "Some patients, though conscious..."
Hippocrates, *Precepts,* chapter 6 (found online at <www.acponline.org/medquotes>).

Page 122: "A competent doctor..."
Jimmie C. Holland, M.D., and Sheldon Lewis, *The Human Side of Cancer* (New York: HarperCollins Publishers Inc., 2000), pp. 55-56.

Page 123: "Research has indicated..."
Geraldine M. Leydon, "Cancer Patients' Information Needs and Information Seeking Behaviour," *British Medical Journal* 320 (April 1, 2000): pp. 909-913.

Page 124: "What you do get..."
Mary-Jo Delvecchio Good, et al, "American Oncology and the Discourse on Hope," *Culture, Medicine and Psychiatry* 14 (1990): p. 67.

Page 125: "Once the tension..."
John Hill, "Living With Cancer: John Hill's Journey," Monroe, Louisiana, *News-Star,* September 29, 2000, p.1B. © 2001 The *News-Star.*

Page 125: "A doctor who treats..."
William Bennett Bean, ed., *Sir William Osler: Aphorisms from His Bedside Teachings and Writings,* collected by Robert Bennett Bean (Springfield, IL: Charles C. Thomas, 1968), p. 53

Page 125: "Explaining and understanding..."
Simpson, Michael, et al, "Doctor-Patient Communication: The Toronto Consensus Statement," *British Medical Journal* 303 (November 30, 1991): p. 1385.

Page 126: "The good physician..."
Francis W. Peabody, M.D., "The Care of the Patient," *Journal of the American Medical Association* 88 (March 19, 1927): pp. 877-882.

Page 128: "the feeling that 'I might...'"
Howard Spiro, et al, eds., *Empathy and the Practice of Medicine* (New Haven, CT: Yale University Press, 1993), p. 2.

Page 130: "Kind words can be..."
Mark Water, compiler, *The New Encyclopedia of Christian Quotations* (Grand Rapids, MI: Baker Books, 2000), p. 556.

Chapter 10—Facing Family and Friends

Page 133: "As long as Moses..."
Exodus 17:11.

Page 134: "I didn't want to..."
John Hill, "Living with Cancer: John Hill's journey," Monroe, Louisiana, *News-Star,* September 1, 2000, p. 3A. © 2001 The *News-Star.*

Page 134: One large study...
P. Reynolds and G.A. Kaplan, "Social Connections and Risk for Cancer: Prospective Evidence from the Alameda County Study," *Behavioral Medicine* 16, no. 3 (Fall 1990): pp. 101-110.

Page 134: Another study done in...
J.S. Goodwin, et al, "The Effect of Marital Status on Stage, Treatment, and Survival of Cancer Patients," *Journal of the American Medical Association* 258, no. 21 (December 4, 1987): pp. 3125-3130.

Page 134: "It can be shown..."
Lea Baider, Cary Cooper, Atara Kaplan De-Nour, eds., *Cancer and the Family* (West Sussex, England: John Wiley & Sons, Ltd., 1996), p. 233.

Page 134: Another study of women...
Nancy Waxler-Morrison, et al, "Effects of Social Relationships on Survival for Women with Breast Cancer: A Prospective Study," *Soc. Sci. Med.* 33, no. 2 (1991): pp. 177-183.

Page 137: "Both our fathers..."
Elizabeth Sherrill, *All the Way to Heaven: An Intimate Faith Journey* (Grand Rapids, MI: Fleming H. Revell Co., 2002), pp. 104-105.

Page 141: "It is almost inconceivable..."
Mary Jo Fisher, M.D., "Live and Learn," *Journal of the American Medical Association* 286, no. 19 (November 21, 2001): p. 2372.

Page 142: "a lifelong empathy with..."
Sherrill, p. 105.

Page 142: "I didn't feel different..."
Alice Stewart Trillin, "Of Dragons and Garden Peas; A Cancer Patient Talks to Doctors," *New England Journal of Medicine* 304 (1981): pp. 699, 700.

Page 143: "human existence..."
Psalm 39:5 NLT.

Page 143: "redoubleth joy..."
Mark Water, compiler, *The New Encyclopedia of Christian Quotations* (Grand Rapids, MI: Baker Books, 2000), p. 387.

Page 145: "Two are better..."
Ecclesiastes 4:9-10.

Chapter 11—Coping with Treatment
Page 147: "I have had enough..."
1 Kings 19:4.

Page 148: "Instead...the angel..."
Marilyn Yocum, "First Aid for Depression," *The Lookout,* Jan. 13, 2002, p. 7.

Page 151: One study done in Germany...
Fernando C. Dimeo, M.D., et al, "Effects of Physical Activity on the Fatigue and Psychologic Status of Cancer Patients During Chemotherapy," *Cancer* 85, no. 10 (May 15, 1999): pp. 2273-2277.

Page 151: "It is clear that lack..."
Maryl L. Winningham, Ph.D., "Strategies for Managing Cancer-Related Fatigue Syndrome: A Rehabilitation Approach," *Cancer* 92, no. 4 (August 15, 2001): p. 991.

Page 154: "Open hands should..."
Elisabeth Elliot, *A Path Through Suffering* (Ann Arbor, MI: Vine Books, 1990), p. 69.

Page 158: "We still live..."
Lewis Sperry Chafer, *Systematic Theology,* vol. 6 (Grand Rapids, MI: Kregel, 1993), p. 295.

Chapter 12—Sensing a Spiritual Dimension

Page 161: "But now that he..."
Herman Melville, *Moby Dick* (Garden City, NY: Dolphin Books), p. 439.

Page 163: "the faith that heals"
As quoted in Walter Larimore, M.D., "Providing Basic Spiritual Care for Patients," *American Family Physician* 63, no. 1 (Jan.1, 2001): p. 40.

Page 163: According to Gallup polls...
As cited in David Larson, M.D., et al, "Patient Spirituality in Clinical Care: Clinical Assessment and Research Findings—Part I," *Primary Care Reports* 6, no. 20 (October 2, 2000): pp. 166-172.

Page 164: "find their master motive..."; "are disposed to use..."
As quoted in Harold Koenig, Michael McCullough, and David Larson, *Handbook of Religion and Health* (New York: Oxford University Press, 2001), pp. 21-22.

Page 164: "What does it mean..."
Jean Fleming, *Finding Focus in a Whirlwind World* (Dallas, TX: Roper Press, 1991), p. 23.

Page 165: One study done in 1991...
As cited in Koenig, p. 310.

Page 165: Another done in 1998...
J. LeBron McBride, PhD, MPH, et al, "The Relationship Between a Patient's Spirituality and Health Experiences," *Family Medicine* 30, no. 2 (February, 1998): pp. 122-126.

Page 166: "You're trying to approach..."
John Sherrill, *They Speak with Other Tongues* (Old Tappan, NJ: Spire Books, 1964), p. 11.

Page 166: "What do they call it..."
Sherrill, p. 11.

Pages 167-168: Three doctors who have...; "Reaching out to..."
Koenig, et al, *Handbook of Religion and Health*, p. 222.

Page 168: "Even when these persons..."; "Religious involvement plays..."
Koenig, et al, *Handbook of Religion and Health*, p. 135.

Page 168: Studies of people with certain...
As cited in Thomas Schwenk, M.D., "Primary Care Management of Depression in Patients with Cancer," *Primary Care & Cancer* 21, no. 1 (January 2001): pp. 47-51.

Page 169: One study of people who were taught..."
F.I. Fawzy, et al, "Malignant Melanoma: Effects of an Early Structured Psychiatric Intervention, Coping and Affective State on Recurrence and Survival 6 Years Later," *Archives of General Psychiatry* 50 (1993): pp. 681-689.

Page 169: "Of those studies, 79..."; "In contrast, persons with no..."; "In many respects, an internalized..."
Koenig, et al *Handbook of Religion and Health*, pp. 101,99,101.

Page 170: "religion as a whole..."
Koenig, et al, p. 153.

Page 170: One study of a group...
Sean O'Laoire, Ph.D., "An Experimental Study of the Effects of Distant, Intercessory Prayer on Self-Esteem, Anxiety, and Depression," *Alternative Therapies* 3, no. 6 (November, 1997): pp. 38-53.

Page 171: "the diagnosis of cancer itself..."; A number of studies show...
Koenig, et al, *Handbook of Religion and Health,* pp. 284,283-284.

Page 171: People who attended once a week...; "The relationship found between..."
Harold Koenig, M.D., et al, "Attendance at Religious Services, Interleukin-6, and Other Biological Parameters of Immune Function in Older Adults," *International Journal of Psychiatry in Medicine* 27, no. 3 (1997): pp. 233-250.

Page 172: "A very high 93 percent..."
James Roberts, et al, "Factors Influencing Views of Patients with Gynecologic Cancer About End-of-Life Decisions," *American Journal of Obstetrics and Gynecology* 176, no. 1 (January, 1997,): pp. 166-172.

Page 172: One study looked at 577...
Harold Koenig, Kenneth Pargament, et al, "Religious Coping and Health Status in Medically Ill Hospitalized Older Adults," *Journal of Nervous and Mental Diseases* 186, no. 9 (September, 1998): pp. 513-521.

Page 173: Another study then reported...
Kenneth Pargament, Harold Koenig, et al, "Religious Struggle as a Predictor of Mortality Among Medically Ill Elderly Patients," *Archives of Internal Medicine* 161 (August 13/27, 2001): pp. 1881-1885. All NLT.

Pages 173-174: "The LORD is close..."; "The LORD is kind and merciful..." "Come to me, all..."; "Give all your worries..."; "Death can't, and life can't..."
Psalm 34:18; Psalm 145:8,13,14,18; Matthew 11:28; 1 Peter 5:7; Romans 8:38-39. All NLT.

Page 174: "There is no pit so deep..."
Corrie ten Boom with John and Elizabeth Sherrill, *The Hiding Place* (Washington Depot, CT: Chosen Books, 1971), p. 197.

Chapter 13—Searching for Meaning

Page 177: "What is left of this girl..."; "At the end of that week..."
Anne Frank, *The Diary of a Young Girl* (New York: Bantam Books, 1993), entry for Tuesday, 7 March, 1944, p. 169.

Page 178: "the prisoner who had lost..."; "giving a lecture..."
Victor E. Frankl, *Man's Search for Meaning* (New York: Washington Square Press, 1985), pp. 94,94-95.

Page 178: "Emotion, which is suffering..."
Frankl, p. 95.

Page 179: "I wrote what..."
John Hill, "Living With Cancer: John Hill's Journey," Monroe, Louisiana, *News-Star,* September 15, 2000, p.1B. © 2001 The *News-Star.*

Page 180: "Once more I was humbled..."
John Hill, "Living With Cancer: John Hill's Journey," Monroe, Louisiana, *News-Star,* November 17, 2000, p.1B. © 2001 The *News-Star.*

Page 181: "I can do all things..."
Philippians 4:13 KJV.

Page 181: Victor Frankl considered...; "There are situations..."
Frankl, pp. 170,137.

Page 182: "You can pray..."; "Having a prayer ministry..."
Dale Matthews, M.D., with Connie Clark, *The Faith Factor: Proof of the Healing Power of Prayer* (New York: Viking, 1998), pp. 139,140.

Page 183: "a Supermeaning..."
Matthew Scully, "Victor Frankl at Ninety: An Interview," *First Things* 52 (April 1995): pp.39-43; accessed at <www.first-things.com/ftissues/ft9504/scully.html>.

Page 183: "Since we are..."
Romans 8:17-18 NLT.

Page 184: In *The Story of Eric Liddell*...
The Story of Eric Liddell (Grand Rapids, MI: RBC Ministries).
Available at <www.dhp.org>.

Page 184: "This interactive relationship..."; "Religious convictions
may..."
Jimmie Holland, et al, "The Role of Religious and Spiritual
Beliefs in Coping with Malignant Melanoma," *Psycho-Oncology* 8 (1999): p. 23.

Page 185: "Smooth seas..."
Mark Water, compiler, *The New Encyclopedia of Christian
Quotations* (Grand Rapids, MI: Baker Books, 2000), p. 19.

Page 186: "Dear brothers and sisters..."
James 1:2-4 NLT.

Page 186: "Life can only be..."
The New Encyclopedia of Christian Quotations, p. 608.

Afterword

Page 190: "because we know..."
Romans 5:3-5.

Page 191: "A clay pot..."
Mildred W. Struven, as quoted in Mark Water, compiler, *The
New Encyclopedia of Christian Quotations* (Grand Rapids, MI:
Baker Books, 2000), p. 984.

A DIFFERENT KIND OF MIRACLE

by *Emilie Barnes*

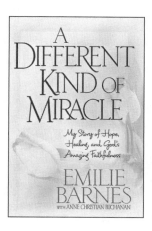

✺

Beloved bestselling author Emilie Barnes covers new, intimate territory in this book based on her life-changing encounter with cancer. A Different Kind of Miracle *illustrates how God's faithfulness and hope are divine gifts, extended to us in the midst of every kind of pain.*

Emilie Barnes' very foundations were shaken when she heard the dreaded word "cancer." But in the long process of treatment, she discovered just how sturdy those Christ-centered foundations were. Here she shares with you what she learned and provides comforting, encouraging words to those who are going through difficulties—be it illness, bereavement, loss, or relationship problems.

As she shares her story, Emilie holds out her hand and says, "Come with me…I'll walk with you along the way." You will find hope and promises of blessings in chapters that talk about…

- ✺ Earthquake Days: what to do when the foundation beneath you shakes

- ✺ The Cupboard's Not Bare: trusting the reality of God's provision

- ✺ Tomorrow Always Dawns: living in hope

If you are experiencing difficulties or wish to understand someone else's pain, *A Different Kind of Miracle* will help you see God's unfailing faithfulness.

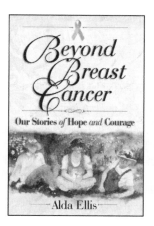

Beyond Breast Cancer

Our Stories of Hope and Courage

Alda Ellis

BEYOND BREAST CANCER
by *Alda Ellis*

When the storms of life wreak unexpected havoc, when a shock comes out of the blue, hope cuts a tiny path of light through the darkness.

Alda Ellis, creator of Alda's Forever bath and body products, lost her own mother to breast cancer. Her passionate concern for women flows from her personal experience and her deeply moving personal interviews with breast cancer survivors. In *Beyond Breast Cancer,* she shares the encouraging and inspirational testimonies of 12 women whose lives have been touched by this devastating disease, such as...

- 39-year-old Debbie, who faced her treatment with the love of friends and a strong sense of faith. Soon after, she created the pink ribbon pin—a symbol of hope recognized across the world.

- Marcia, a young wife and mother, who faced two different cancers in 11 years. To the women she now encourages as a volunteer, her life is living proof that breast cancer is not a death sentence, but can add meaning and purpose to life.

For women who struggle with breast cancer—and for friends, families, and caregivers of breast cancer patients—these uplifting stories will create a portrait of courage vivid with faith, encouragement, and the gift of hope.